This Common
Secret

This Common Secret

*My Journey
as an Abortion Doctor*

Susan Wicklund

with *Alan Kesselheim*

PublicAffairs
New York

Published in the United States by PublicAffairs™, a member of the Perseus Books Group.

Printed in the United States of America.

PublicAffairs books are available at special discounts for bulk purchases in the U.S. by corporations, institutions, and other organizations. For more information, please contact the Special Markets Department at the Perseus Books Group, 2300 Chestnut Street, Suite 200, Philadelphia, PA 19103, or call (800) 255-1514, or email special.markets@perseusbooks.com.

BOOK DESIGN BY JEFF WILLIAMS

Library of Congress Cataloging-in-Publication Data

Wicklund, Susan.
This common secret : my journey as an abortion doctor / Susan Wicklund with Alan Kesselheim. — 1st ed.
    p. cm.
Includes bibliographical references.
ISBN-13: 978-1-58648-480-4 (hardcover)
ISBN-10: 1-58648-480-X (hardcover)
1. Wicklund, Susan. 2. Physicians—United States—Biography. 3. Abortion—United States. I. Kesselheim, Alan S., 1952- II. Title.

[DNLM: 1. Wicklund, Susan. 2. Physicians, Women—United States—Biography. 3. Abortion, Legal—United States—Biography. 4. Abortion, Legal—history—United States. 5. History, 20th Century—United States. 6. History, 21st Century—United States. WZ 100 W6375 2007]

R154.W47A3 2007
610.92—dc22
[B]
                                                              2007016594

First Edition

10 9 8 7 6 5 4 3 2 1

In honor of all the clinic staff, doctors, volunteers, and escorts who routinely brave harassment and personal attack in order to make sure that American women can continue to freely exercise their reproductive rights.

contents

This Common
Secret

A woman's life can really be a succession
of lives, each revolving around some emotionally
compelling situation or challenge, and each
marked off by some intense experience.

WALLIS SIMPSON
DUCHESS OF WINDSOR
(1896–1986)

chapter one

When I drove into Grandma's driveway, all I could think about was how she would react. I had started out to tell her many times over the last few years. On so many visits I had meant to have that conversation but had never found a way. Something had always intervened. Some other errand had always come up. I had found a way not to face her judgment.

It didn't matter that I was rock solid in my resolve and in my chosen profession. This was my grandma. My Flower Grandma. What she thought of me mattered a lot, and I had no idea how she'd take it.

It was February of 1992, a Saturday afternoon. The next day the *60 Minutes* segment I'd done with Lesley Stahl would air. Grandma never missed *60 Minutes*. I had to tell her before she saw it—before she saw her oldest granddaughter talking about the death threats and stalking and personal harassment my family and I were enduring.

The harassment wasn't the issue that mattered now. It was the fact that I was, as a physician, traveling to five clinics in three states to provide abortion services for as many as one hundred women every week, and that I had been doing this work for four years already.

I wasn't at all ashamed of my career. In fact, I always considered it an honor to be involved in reproductive choices, this most personal and intimate realm for women. I just never felt the need to make it public. Very few of my family and friends were aware of what I did.

Within a day, however, everyone I had grown up with, everyone who knew my family, and every member of my family would know the truth. Would I be isolated and ostracized? Would I get support or condemnation?

I pulled off the highway and into the drive leading to the house I'd grown up in. Mom and Dad still lived in the white, two-story, wood-frame home.

Dad had worked as a precision machinist in the town of Grantsburg, ten miles away. His love had been the gunsmithing, hunting, and fishing he did in his free time. My three siblings and I had always been included. We were as competent with firearms, field dressing a deer, or catching a batch of sunfish as anyone in the area. Dad was retired now and not feeling well. It was painful to watch him, the strong man who starred in my memories, struggling with simple tasks.

Mom was retired too, from her elected position as clerk of court for our county. She was the one everyone—especially women—turned to for advice and support. Mom had been instrumental, many years earlier, in starting a shelter for victims of domestic abuse. In her job she had seen so many situations in which women and children had nowhere to go for help. It was just like Mom to tackle a need that everyone else ignored.

I grew up in the unincorporated village of Trade Lake, Wisconsin, a small gathering of about six houses, several of which were the homes of my relatives. The only business left was one small gas station/grocery store. When I was a kid, there had been a feed store and creamery and a meat market, but those had been gone for better than thirty years. Only rotten shells of buildings remained.

Even now, Trade Lake is a very rural place. People still raise chickens in backyards, drive tractors to the little grocery store. Chimneys puff wood smoke in the winter.

The small river that wound its way through our yard came into view. Behind it were the woods where I'd built forts and climbed oak trees with my sister. She and I each had a horse and spent the bulk of our summers out of doors. Grandma and Grandpa had lived just down the road. We picked mayflowers every spring with Grandma. In the summer we fished with Grandpa for sunfish and crappies using cane poles baited with worms dug out of the garden.

Mine had been a good childhood. This was a safe place. Turning into the driveway had always been a good thing—a coming home. This time was different.

I felt myself sweating under my coat. My racing heart pushed against my throat. I had to reveal something to my dear grandma that could change everything she believed and loved about me.

Grandma had moved into a trailer house in the backyard of the family home. Grandpa had died fifteen years earlier, and Mom wanted her mother even closer—just steps across the yard. I saw the clothesline hung with rugs, the twine still strung up on the porch to hold the morning glories that filled the railings in the summer.

Flower Grandma. My daughter, Sonja, gave her the name when she was three and there were too many grandmas to keep track of. Sonja spent many days baking cookies with her great-grandmother and playing outside, just as I had as a young girl. She ran back and forth constantly between the houses of her two grandmothers. This grandma always had flowers growing in every nook and cranny, inside and out.

Flower Grandma she became, and Flower Grandma she stayed. Before long my entire extended family called her Flower Grandma, and even her friends at the local senior center fell into the habit.

I coasted to a stop at the bottom of the slope. I sat there long enough to take a deep breath and fight back a few unexpected tears. I didn't know where the sadness came from. The car engine ticked. I was alone, vulnerable, aching. Was I longing for those simple childhood days, whipping down the hill on my sled? How far I'd come from that.

I peeled myself out of the car, shed my coat, and left it on the seat. It was unusually warm for February in Wisconsin. The hardwood forest was all bare sticks and hard lines. I knew it would soon be time to tap the maple trees and cook the syrup we all loved on Grandma's Swedish pancakes.

I turned and deliberately moved up the steps to the trailer house. I was terrified of what Grandma would say, but there was no avoiding this moment.

The big door was already open by the time I got to the top step. Out peeked her welcoming smile. She was giggling.

"Hi, Grandma!"

"Oh my goodness! What a surprise! What a sweet, sweet surprise! Did I know you were coming today?"

I hugged her in the doorway, held her tight, stepped inside.

"Did you somehow know I was making ginger snaps?" she teased as she set a plate full on the kitchen table. She poured me a glass of milk, and I sat down on the wooden chair next to hers. I tried to bury myself in the smell of her place, a mixture of ginger cookies, Estée Lauder perfume (the one in the blue hourglass bottle always on her dresser), and home permanents. She and Mom always gave each other perms, trying to get just the right curl in their hair. The smell never left the place.

I think she sensed that I had come to talk about something important. I started talking a few times about other, inconsequential things; then, finally, I plunged in.

"Grandma, you know I work as a doctor."

"Of course. And we are all so proud of you."

"Yes, but I don't think you know the whole story. I'm a doctor who works mostly for women, helping women with pregnancy problems."

Flower Grandma hesitated just a second, pushed back her chair, stood, and held out her hand for me to follow. She went to sit in her rocker, the same one sitting in my living room today. The rocker I have sat in so many hours since. The rocker I sit in right now, writing this down and trembling as I do.

She seemed distant. I moved to the old leather hassock beside her. She took my hand and placed it on top of one of hers, then covered it with her other one. Our hands made a stack on the arm of the rocker—old skin, young skin. We sat in silence a minute. She turned to look directly at me.

Her eyes, framed by gentle wrinkles, were full of some deep trouble.

After a moment, she stared straight ahead and started to speak. Slowly. Deliberately. In a very quiet voice. At the same time she began stroking my hand. It was as if the gentle stroking was pushing her to talk.

"When I was sixteen years old, my best friend got pregnant," she said. A chill went through me.

"I always believed it was her father that was using her," she went on, "but I never knew for sure. She came to my sister, Violet, and me, and asked us to help her."

While I listened, thoughts whirled through my head. Stories I had read of women self-aborting and dying of infections when a safe, legal option was not available. The women who came to the clinics where I worked, many of whom still had to overcome huge difficulties to end an unwanted pregnancy.

It isn't uncommon to have patients confide in me that prior to coming in for an abortion, they had used combinations of herbs to try to force a miscarriage. These home remedies can be extremely dangerous and have caused the deaths of many women.

I felt myself tighten and withdraw, anticipating what Flower Grandma was going to tell me. I wanted to see her eyes, but she kept them straight ahead. And she kept stroking my hand. So soft. I only wanted to think about those hands. Hands embracing and caressing mine—strong, gentle, soft.

"The three of us were so naïve. We knew very little about these things, but we had heard that if you put something long and sharp 'up there,' in the private place, sometimes it would end the pregnancy."

In spite of myself I conjured the modest room: a dresser in the corner with a kerosene lamp and maybe a hairbrush or hand mirror beside it. I saw three young, scared girls, still children, acting on old wives' tales and whispered instructions.

My stomach turned. Was this my grandma? Was I really here in her trailer house hearing this? I could barely breathe. She kept talking, all the while stroking the top of my hand, her eyes looking off into space, traveling back in time. Occasionally a pat-pat with her hand would break the rhythm of the stroking. Such old skin, full of brown age spots and paper thin. Stroking my hand in perfect measure with her words.

Please just stop, Grandma. Don't tell me anymore. Just hold my hand, and let's talk about what you'll plant in the spring. Tell me about the oatmeal bread you baked yesterday. Are there many birds coming to the bird feeder? I was flushed all over. And still she stroked while she talked. Pat-pat, stroke.

"We closed ourselves, the three of us, in one of the bedrooms late one morning. We didn't talk much, and she didn't ever cry out in pain. It took a few tries to make the blood come. None of us spoke. We didn't know what to expect next, or what to do when the blood kept coming. It was all over the sheets. All over us. So bright red. It was awful. It just wouldn't stop."

She was still stroking my hand. I was shaking uncontrollably. I stared at the African violets under the plant light, trying to make them the focus of my attention. Her voice was a monotone, never a pause.

"We put rags inside of her to try to stop the bleeding, but they soaked full. We all three stayed in her bed. We just didn't know what to do."

My hand was trembling so hard it was all I could do to keep it on top of hers. She grasped it briefly, held it tight, patted it a few times, and then went on.

"We stayed there together, unable to move, even after she was dead. Her father found us, all three of us, in the bed. He stood in the doorway, staring. No words for a long time. When he did speak, he told my sister and me to leave and that we were never, ever to speak of this. We were not to tell anyone, ever. Ever."

She stopped stroking my hand and sat still before turning to look directly at me. "That was seventy-two years ago. You are the first person I have ever told that story. I am still so ashamed of what happened. We were just so young and scared. We didn't know anything."

Terrible sadness welled up inside me. And anger. I couldn't picture my grandma as someone responsible for the death of anything, much less her best friend at the age of sixteen. She had carried this secret all her life, kept it inside, festering with guilt and shame.

I wondered if the pregnancy was indeed the result of incest. Would it have made a difference? What were friends and family told about the death? What had they actually used to start the bleeding? What had the doctor put on the death certificate as the cause of death?

I knew, through the patients I had met, that no one has to look very far into their family history to find these stories tucked away, hidden from view. But it didn't lessen the shock of finding it here, so close, in the heart of my own family.

Flower Grandma sighed and held my hand tight. Tears welled in her eyes.

"I know exactly what kind of work you do, and it is a good thing. People like you do it safely so that people like me don't murder their best friends. I told you how proud I am of what you do, and I meant it."

» In 1930, illegal abortions were recorded
as the cause of death for 2,700 women,
18 percent of all maternal deaths in that year.

» Before 1973 and the passage of
Roe v. Wade, an estimated 1.2 million women
had illegal abortions in the United States yearly.
As many as 5,000 died each year as a result.

» Between 1973 and 2002, more than
42 million legal abortions were performed.

» Risk of death during childbirth is eleven times
higher than the risk of death from legal abortion.

chapter two

Flower Grandma is gone now. So is my mother. I can share the story my grandmother kept inside from the time she was a young girl. Her story and hundreds of others like it desperately need to be told. We need their legacy so we don't forget, and to remind ourselves that every family has a similar tale somewhere in its history.

It has been my privilege and honor to hear many women's stories and to participate in their unfolding. As a young woman, the idea that I might be in such a position would have seemed far-fetched indeed. No, actually, it would have seemed impossible.

In April 1980 I was a twenty-six-year-old mom living in Wisconsin, raising a daughter alone, working part-time at a VFW bar and part-time in a natural foods co-op. I was on welfare, medical assistance, and food stamps. My post–high school education consisted of a handful of community college classes, none of which fit together or qualified me for anything, with one exception.

I had given birth to my daughter at home just north of San Francisco, where her father and I were living. To prepare for the event, I took birthing classes, which led to an interest in midwifery. Since Sonja's birth, I had been involved in many births, both in homes and in hospitals, volunteering as an advocate for women in labor.

I knew from my own experience how empowering it was for women to be informed. With that information, women feel secure about expressing their needs. Their active participation changes the entire dynamic. I loved the energy of those births. By the late 1970s, however, midwives were being prosecuted for practicing medicine without a license, so I had resorted to teaching birth classes in an effort to optimize the hospital experience for women.

Sonja's dad, David, and I had gone our separate ways, having fundamental differences in lifestyles. I had yearned for the rural life again and wanted Sonja to grow up knowing her grandparents. David was a jazz musician who needed and craved the big city life. When it came down to it, I couldn't live on the road following a musician around, and he couldn't imagine a life full of chopping wood and hunting deer. Our breakup had been amicable, and David continued to be very committed to Sonja even after I moved back to the Midwest in 1979.

On Easter Sunday 1980 I was invited to a gathering of people on the West Bank of Minneapolis. The host roasted a lamb in an open pit and provided traditional Greek wine. It was the first really warm day of spring. I was wearing a piecework skirt I had sewn, a pink V-necked T-shirt, and Birkenstock sandals. I fit right in. Sonja, nearly three, was having a blast running around with all the other kids.

I began talking with a man perhaps twenty years older than I. We sat on the grass drinking red wine and soaking up sunshine. An occasional dog streaked through the chaos.

It was one of those conversations that avoided the common superficialities. Hal questioned me about my interests and skills and background. He wanted to know what made me happy, what frustrated me. Did I like travel, or was I a homebody? He wanted me to tell him about Sonja's birth and about the training I had as a midwife. He asked about what I liked to read. What my parents did. What my fears were, and my dreams.

I told him how much I loved the contact with women and what satisfaction I got from teaching birthing classes. I felt I could communicate the information effectively and in a way most of the women understood. My collection of books on pregnancy and birth and midwifery and early childhood development was growing rapidly, and I was devouring them. I missed the chance to be involved in home births now that I was back in the Midwest.

I also talked about my dreams of somehow making a difference, a real difference, in peoples' lives. I didn't know what or how or when that might happen, but I knew I would not be content to work in the local grocery store or VFW all my life. I wanted more diversity. More challenge. More adventure.

It seemed as if we'd been there most of the afternoon when Hal looked at me and said, "It is clear that you need to go to medical school. You would be a great doctor."

"*Me?!* Be a doctor?"

I hugged myself across my belly, tipping over into the grass and laughing until I cried. He had to be out of his mind! Sonja came running up and jumped on me. I curled up tighter, still laughing.

The idea was preposterous. The logistics alone would be impossible.

We went on with the day, enjoying the sunshine and good food and music. Local musicians kept pulling out instruments and playing them late into the night. It was only much later that I learned Hal worked as a career counselor at a nearby federal prison.

Crazy as it was, in the weeks following the party, Hal's suggestion kept echoing in my thoughts. I knew my life was on hold, waiting for some nudge, some direction. By mid-May, Sonja and I had moved into a tent in a goat pasture. We were helping some friends with a building project. Living right on site seemed like a good idea.

Summer went on, full of building fences, tending gardens, moving rocks for a foundation, but the seed Hal had planted that Easter Sunday wouldn't go away. The idea of college and then medical school seemed far out of my reach. I had absolutely no money to pay for tuition or child care for Sonja. I didn't know if I could even handle the academic challenges. Imagining myself in the role of a doctor was outrageous.

The biggest mental and emotional hurdle I was struggling with was wrapped up in becoming part of the medical community. True, my childhood family doctor had always been kind, someone I looked up to. But he was almost a neighbor, and he was a man. Men were doctors. Women were nurses.

That stereotype wasn't insurmountable, but there was something else I had to deal with. Something much more visceral and daunting. The memory of my own abortion, in 1976, in Portland, Oregon.

When I became pregnant, politics and *Roe v. Wade* were the furthest things from my consciousness. I didn't engage with the political and social issues.

At that time I rented a house with four roommates, including David. I had no money and juggled three jobs: waitressing, cleaning horse stalls, and growing alfalfa sprouts. David played local gigs with jazz musicians in bars and clubs. No part of me was ready to be a mother, and I felt no emotional connection to the pregnancy. I learned from a community health clinic that I could get an abortion just blocks from where I lived.

I called the clinic and made an appointment, but learned that the abortion cost $350, an impossible amount of money, more than I made in a month. All of my roommates pitched in to help me come up with the necessary cash.

The doctor's office was on the second floor of a large building. David came with me. Protesters outside carried signs, tried to talk to us. I was so preoccupied, so anxious, that I only remember them as an annoyance, a hassle.

The first thing they wanted in the tiny office was my money. Pay in advance, all of it, in cash. I was so frightened and unaware. What was supposed to happen? No counseling took place, no explanation of procedures or options; no one tried to understand my circumstances or answer my questions.

In another tiny room a nurse told me to undress and lie down on the table.

"What are you doing?" I wanted to know.

"Just be still," she said. She sat in front of me and put a cold speculum into my vagina. I could feel tugging and pulling, but no real pain. She was done quickly, took out the speculum, and then told me to get dressed.

"Am I done?" I asked.

"Done?" she slapped the words at me. "No. I just put something into your cervix that will make it open up for the abortion. You should leave now and come back at three this afternoon."

I still had no idea what to expect.

"What's happening?" David kept asking when we left. "What are they going to do?" I couldn't deal with his questions. I had no answers. I had been told nothing, knew only that I had to hold on to my resolve until this was over.

I dropped David off at the house and drove on in our VW bus to work for a few hours, spraying flats of alfalfa seeds and bagging sprouts. I kept cramping, fighting against the pain and anxiety that threatened to overwhelm me. The time dragged.

When we returned, the same woman took me back to the small room, again had me get undressed, and used the speculum to examine me. She removed something she had put inside me earlier, but was impatient with me when I asked questions.

I was moved into a much larger room. It seemed huge, filled with machines and trays of exposed instruments and syringes and needles. Two other women came in. They had me strip naked, lie on a table, and put my feet in stirrups. They put a paper sheet over my upper body and told me to lie still. Then all three of them walked out. No advice, no preparatory explanation, no squeeze of the hand. For a long time I lay there in that vast, cold room, utterly exposed and as vulnerable as I'd ever been in my life.

Finally, the door opened, and a very large man, the doctor, came toward me. I remember looking down over my legs at him, aware of how physically exposed I was.

He said nothing, didn't even tell me his name, asked no questions, but abruptly started to work. An emotional claustrophobia enveloped me. I could feel myself starting to panic.

"What are you doing?" I asked. "Please tell me what you are doing!"

I could feel instruments inside me, a harsh invasion and pain I hadn't expected. "Is it supposed to hurt?" I pleaded.

"Shut up and lie still!" His voice was rough, angry, as if I had no right to intrude. I started to squirm away from him, trying to make him stop long enough to talk to me.

"Please," I pleaded. "Please just tell me what you are doing. Stop. Talk to me. Please!"

He called for nurses to come hold me down.

The claustrophobia grew and grew, the pain kept coming, and I writhed and fought as nurses grabbed my arms and shoulders. I heard myself scream. Tears ran past my ears and into my hair. Then they injected something into my arm, and I faded away from the nightmare.

When I woke, my face was stuck to a Naugahyde couch. I was in a very small room, alone. I struggled up groggily and went to the door. Locked. Panic rose up again, but all I could do was sit and cry until someone let me out.

"If you have problems, go to an emergency room," was the sum total of advice I was given as I went out the door.

Something terrible had been done to me. I felt abused and violated and beaten. I did not feel that I had made a bad choice, that I had done a bad thing. But I knew something bad had been done to me. All I wanted, then, was to escape.

I remember sitting on the dark staircase in our house that weekend and calling my mother, telling her what had happened. "I wish I could be with you," she kept saying. I could hear her voice tremble over the phone, almost two thousand miles away. I wished I had talked to her earlier. I wished I had allowed her to support and comfort me.

After David and I were married and had moved to California, I became pregnant again. He was still playing sax, and I was waitressing, but this time was different. As much as I hadn't felt attached to the earlier pregnancy, this time I felt an immediate connection. I knew I wanted this baby.

My problem, and it grew more and more worrisome as the pregnancy advanced, was that I was terrified of doctors and clinics and hospitals. My abortion experience had scarred me. I simply couldn't relinquish control over my body to someone who might treat me as badly as I had been treated in Portland. The thought of being in a sterile hospital room with my feet in stirrups and no one I loved nearby was horrifying.

Friends talked about the possibility of having a home birth with a midwife. As soon as it sank in that this was a real alternative, I jumped on it. The connection I made with our midwife, Nan, was immediate and wonderful.

The pregnancy and the birth were both completely normal. In stark contrast to my abortion experience, during

Sonja's birth I was surrounded by people I loved and who loved me. I was in my own bed, in my own home, the tiny apartment we rented. And I knew exactly what was happening, both because of my own research and because my questions were honored and answered.

Desperate Measures
Used to End Unwanted Pregnancies:

» use of sharp object like
  coat hanger or knitting needle

» scalding water baths

» massive doses of herbal concoctions,
  such as black cohosh teas

» douches with lye,
  cleaning fluids, boiling water

» excessive exercise

— chapter three

Now, three years after Sonja's home birth, I was considering the possibility of entering a medical career, a profession that held real terror for me, as well as fascination and challenge. It would mean I could attend home births as a physician and educate women about alternatives. It would mean that I could support Sonja.

Since the breakup of my marriage, providing for Sonja had become a major preoccupation and necessity. I knew that public assistance was a temporary boost, but I didn't want that to become my permanent solution.

In the end, what tipped the scales was the realization that if I actually pulled this off, I could make sure my patients were treated differently than I had been—with respect and decency. The memory of my own abortion troubled me, but it also hardened my resolve. I refused to let one bad doctor dictate a decision over my life direction.

By the beginning of July going to college was sounding like a challenge I wanted to accept. I made a trip to the University of Wisconsin at River Falls and went to the financial aid office to see what the possibilities might be. I was greeted by encouraging, knowledgeable people who helped me through the landscape of forms and formalities needed to apply for college and for student loans.

I enrolled in August. I hadn't declared any long-term intention, but I was at least going to get started. Sonja and I gave up our wall tent and moved two hours south, into a trailer house next to the river just blocks from campus. Our first morning I set her in a red Radio Flyer wagon piled high with books and extra clothes and snacks. I dropped her off at the day care on campus and began college full-time.

My declared major was sociology. I still didn't know if I could handle the hard sciences. I hadn't studied physics or chemistry in high school. How dare I have the audacity to think I could even *be* a doctor?

The first quarter was all it took to boost my confidence. I took chemistry and math, along with biology, psychology, and English, and came out with a 4.0 GPA. By the end of the first year I was on a roll and loving every bit of it. I went to summer school to do the equivalent of a year's worth of physics and continued with excellent grades and increasing optimism.

Sonja went with me everywhere. In warm weather I pulled her around campus in the red wagon. During the winter months she burrowed into a nest of blankets in a box mounted on a sled. She came with me to biology lab and counted fruit flies through the dissecting scope. She loved the poster of the human skeleton and learned the names of all the bones with me. When she fell off the porch and broke her arm, she walked beside me into the emergency room holding her arm.

"I think it's the radius," she told the doctor, and she was right.

The second winter we lived in a drafty farmhouse outside of town. It had no running water, and our electricity was limited to one extension cord that ran in the door from a junction box outside, but it was rent-free. The owners wanted someone there to keep vandals out. Every evening Sonja would sit on the couch, cuddled up in a sleeping bag and cutting out paper snowflakes, while I built a fire in the wood stove. I would stoke that stove for hours, using the wood my father and sister had hauled down from home, 120 miles away. Even at that, it was all I could do to get the heat up to fifty degrees. By the end of winter, every inch of wall space was covered in paper snowflakes.

But I was happy being a student. Chemistry, biology, physics, all the course work I had feared—from photosynthesis to physics in everyday life, I kept having ah-hah! moments. I aced course after course.

I was happy, too, because I'd met a man named Randy. Actually, I'd known Randy slightly back in high school. He had been a senior when I was a freshman, and I remembered him for his successful crusade to abolish the student dress code. We met again when I was home visiting and working at the local food co-op. He was working as a heavy equipment operator.

We started spending weekends together whenever possible. I loved Randy's genuine honesty, his dependability, and his solid commitment to people and the causes he believed in. He was the only person I trusted with my true medical aspirations.

Most important, Randy fell head over heels in love with Sonja. The feeling was mutual. Almost from the start, Sonja started calling Randy "Randad."

It wasn't until I'd finished two years of school, and was fueled with newfound confidence, that I felt able to articulate my ultimate goal to my family and friends: I was going to be a doctor.

My mother was encouraging and proud and promised to do all she could to help. There was no money to help with expenses, but she could pitch in with child care. My father was skeptical but knew enough not to say it out loud. Maybe he was worried about where he'd have to haul wood to next. I could feel the sideways looks of aunts, uncles, and cousins, very few of whom had gone past high school.

Higher education had never been a part of our extended family expectations. Mom would have loved to go to college and law school, but the times and circumstances did not allow it. Dad had only finished eighth grade, but he had enrolled in machinist school on the GI bill after serving in World War II. He had earned a GED many years later, along with some of his brothers. Dad and all five of his brothers served in the war.

After three years I earned my bachelor of science degree in biology and was accepted into medical school. Another move for Sonja, but this time we joined a married couple with two kids. The husband was in the same program I was, and the wife was in nursing school. We shared childcare responsibilities, along with meals and bedtime stories. And, as Sonja pointed out, you just had to turn up the thermostat to make it warmer.

Most weekends we drove down to be with Randy. I studied nonstop, but Randy and Sonja had their standard routine. They'd make a trip to the dump, buy groceries, do chores, then head off on the round of family visits to grandmas and aunts and uncles. Randy built Sonja a sandbox in the yard, where she played for hours.

It didn't take long in medical school to see that even though women were allowed in, it was a system run by and for men. Most of the lecturers and attending physicians were men. All the deans and department heads were men.

There were times when it was all I could do to keep my mouth shut. Other times I was not able to contain myself and took actions that almost got me expelled. One incident that put me toe to toe with the medical school hierarchy still makes me shudder.

It was the first morning of a third-year medical student rotation in obstetrics and gynecology. We met in a lecture hall for a discussion of pelvic anatomy with the attending physician. He told us that the best way to learn pelvic anatomy was to do an exam on a relaxed pelvis and that a woman under general anesthesia was ideal. We were led to the operating room suite and were told we would all be performing pelvic exams on five or six women and then discussing our findings.

It dawned on me that these were women admitted for a variety of operations or procedures. A gallbladder surgery, perhaps, or breast lumpectomy or knee surgery. I suspected that the patients hadn't been told they would be undergoing pelvic exams by eight or ten medical students while under general anesthesia.

My suspicion was confirmed. I was absolutely appalled and walked up to confront the attending physician.

"So we're all doing pelvic exams on this patient?" I asked.

"Yes."

"Without her permission?"

He stared at me.

"We're all really supposed to do this?"

"Quit asking questions," he said. "Scrub in and get with the program."

I refused, turned around, and went directly to the department head.

"I can't believe we are expected to do this," I said. "It is a terrible violation."

"These women have come to a teaching hospital," he replied. "They understand that medical students are present and need to learn. They'll never know it anyway."

"Are you proud of this teaching institution?"

"Of course," he replied.

"Then you'll have no problem when I go to the local paper and discuss this teaching practice."

I knew very well that this could mean the end of my medical education, but if this was what it meant to become a doctor, I had no desire to go any further. After a heated discussion, the department head agreed to put a halt to pelvic exams on anesthetized women, and I agreed not to go to the papers with the story.

In spite of the fact that almost half of the women in this country have an abortion at some time in their reproductive lives, abortion was not acknowledged, discussed, or described during my ob-gyn rotation. When I asked to be taught the procedure, I was met with total resistance. It was simply not a program option. This refusal only made me more determined.

Shouldn't a physician be able to at least intelligently discuss all the options for women with unplanned pregnancies?

I was finally able to arrange, on my own, an elective reproductive health rotation at another institution. There I was able to learn about the various methods of abortion and observe procedures.

Memories of my own abortion kept creeping in, memories too painful to talk about, but I had been in enough medical situations by then to realize that my experience was not the norm. I was anxious to see how procedures were done in a legitimate, well-run clinic.

The first abortion I saw during that rotation was for a woman who was halfway through her pregnancy. The fetus had an abnormality incompatible with life. It had started out as a very planned and wanted pregnancy. When the abnormality was diagnosed through an ultrasound, the woman chose to end the pregnancy instead of going full-term, delivering the baby, and having it die immediately.

Most abortions done at this stage are for similar reasons, or to save the life of the mother, but knowing the circumstances did not soften the visual reality of a twenty-one-week fetus. Seeing an arm being pulled through the vaginal canal was shocking. One of the nurses in the room escorted me out when the color left my face.

Not only was it a visceral shock; this was something I had to think deeply about.

I had been about eight weeks pregnant when I had my abortion. I knew from my embryology classes in the first year of medical school that an eight-week embryo is about the size of my thumbnail. It cannot feel pain or think or have any sense of being. I have never regretted that abortion.

Confronting a twenty-one-week fetus is very different. It still cannot feel pain or think or have any sense of being, but the reality is, this cannot be called "tissue." It was not something I could be comfortable with. From that moment, I chose to limit my abortion practice to the first trimester: fourteen weeks or less.

Over the next six weeks I met eight to ten women in the clinic almost every day, women who had come to end pregnancies for a variety of reasons. For some it was financially motivated. Others had educations to finish or careers they had just started. Some were in abusive relationships and did not want that connection to the man. There were women with chronic illnesses whose lives would be in jeopardy if the pregnancy continued. And there were women carrying fetuses with genetic abnormalities or anomalies incompatible with life. Many had been using a form of birth control that failed.

Never once did these decisions seem easy or casual. Every one was the product of tremendous personal struggle. Anyone who claims otherwise is either very ignorant or un-kind or both. Anyone who says that women use abortion as a method of birth control or as a simple matter of convenience should spend a day in a clinic where abortions are per-formed. No honest person would ever make that statement again.

Equally important and revealing is the fact that women who have abortions come from every level of education, every income bracket, and every age from puberty to menopause. They are Catholic and Jewish, Protestant and Buddhist, ag-nostic and atheist. Every race and every ethnic group. Every possible woman. They are, in truth, our sisters, aunts, grand-mothers, music teachers, neighbors, and best friends.

By the end of six weeks I had become steadfast in my be-lief that abortion has to be legal and available for all women, even when the pregnancy is into the second trimester. Women cannot be forced to bear children they are unable to care for physically, financially, or emotionally. Women cannot be forced to continue with a pregnancy that may cost them their lives. The bottom line, as expressed by my friend Liz Karlin, is, "Women have abortions because they want to be good mothers."

What struck home more than anything during that rota-tion was how drastic and tragic it would be to have this choice taken away from women. By the end of it, I had learned that abortions could be performed with compassion and respect, just as I had suspected. It was an experience I had been denied, but one I vowed not to deny any woman who became my patient.

From there I went on to another elective rotation in Salt Lake City, Utah, to study infertility, in vitro fertilization, and embryo transfer. It might initially seem strange for a doctor who wants to do abortions to enroll in both those rotations. But true choice is a matter of understanding and weighing all the options, and then being free to carry out the most appropriate one.

While I was leaning toward a specialty in some aspect of women's reproductive health, I was still weighing other options. I found genetics fascinating, for instance, and was intrigued by the career possibilities in forensic pathology.

Before I had learned to do abortions and was still early in my training, I met a woman whose circumstances illustrated the life-and-death reality of choice. I didn't know it then, but her case would be the turning point in my medical career.

When I encountered her, I was one of many students, interns, and doctors doing prenatal care in a low-income clinic. Most of my time was spent getting initial information from patients, keeping charts, taking medical histories—the grunt work of the process.

This woman, when I first saw her, wouldn't look at me directly. She seemed heavy with defeat. She moved slowly and spoke slowly. I was the first person in the system she had seen. I began working on her chart, getting her ready for the exam. "I can't have this baby," she blurted out.

"What do you mean?"

"I can't have it," her voice was hushed, frightened. "He'll kill it if I do."

"Who? Who will kill it?"

"My man. The county already took my two girls because he beat them. I already lost my two girls. I can't lose another. He'll kill it. I know he will!" She was looking at me now, beseeching, her voice strident.

"Have you had counseling?" She shook her head. "There are shelters for abused women. Places you can get help, where you can get away from him." She kept shaking her head.

"I can't have this baby. He'll kill it."

I began making inquiries over the next few days. The social service agencies were aware of the case, knew the history, but couldn't be mobilized. They wouldn't agree to take the child after birth until there was evidence of abuse. The woman had no money. $350 for an abortion might as well have been $350,000.

When I saw her again, I asked her about adoption, but she adamantly refused.

I felt completely helpless. This woman's predicament seemed insurmountable. The rest of the medical personnel in the clinic were no help. I saw her periodically throughout her pregnancy. Eventually she stopped pleading with me, but in her eyes I read deep fear and reproach. I was her first connection to the clinic, the one she chose to confide in, a person she thought had real power, and I was impotent.

The night she delivered was incredibly busy on labor and delivery. I scurried from patient to patient, prepping, comforting, coaching, assisting doctors. Her birth was one of many, an uncomplicated procedure lost in the confusion of a hectic night. Her "man" was not there. She had no visitors.

When we sent her and the baby on their way in a taxi two days later, she wouldn't meet my eyes.

"Be safe," I said, as I closed the cab door. She rode away, out of my life. I thought about her from time to time, but things careened on. Only the present demands stayed in focus.

Nearly a week later my pager went off, and all I could hear was my name and the words "emergency room." When I walked through the swinging doors, there she was again. I saw her holding her infant son. ER staff surrounded her, trying to get her to hand over the baby, but she was holding the limp body tightly.

When she saw me, she held it out, shaking with emotion. "It's your fault!" she cried. The baby, this infant, just born and already dead, lay across her arms like an accusation. "It should never have been born." The woman's face was twisted in anguish and hatred. "It's your fault."

I stood with my hand over my mouth, frozen in place. Now I was the one unable to meet her eyes. I felt a surge of mingled guilt and frustration and anger. Guilt for not being more persistent in finding her the help she had asked for. Frustration with a system that doesn't protect the weakest

— 32 —

and poorest and most vulnerable. Anger at the father for all the obvious reasons. I also felt utterly inadequate.

For a long time I felt it was indeed my fault. Her face haunted me. Her words echoed in my head. Even now her face still confronts me. At that moment I knew with absolute certainty that I had to learn to do safe, legal abortions. I had to be able to offer that service to my own patients. Abortion is about life: quality of life for infants, children, and adults. Everywhere and in every sense of the word. Life, not death.

The self is not something ready-made,
but something in continuous
formation through choice of action.

—JOHN DEWEY (1859–1952)

— chapter four

Just weeks before my graduation from medical school in 1987, Randy and I were married in a private ceremony. Two good friends, Sonja, and Flower Grandma were the only people in attendance. Then, after graduation, we held a huge family party to celebrate both events. My parents were embarrassingly proud. I remember dancing with Dad to the "Blue Skirt Waltz," closing my eyes and pretending I was ten years old again. Within days we were packing up for my ob-gyn internship in Portland, Oregon.

Before we left, though, I had one stop to make in St. Paul. I tracked down Hal, the man who had first put the crazy notion in my head that I could be a doctor.

Coming up his front porch steps, I wasn't sure that he would even remember me. His broad grin and open arms reassured me that he had not forgotten the hippy mom on a bright afternoon more than seven years earlier. His eyes asked the question, and my nod gave the answer. I made it! I was a doctor! This man whom I had only met once in my life had changed everything for me.

We sat on his front porch. He wanted all the details. I told him Sonja was now ten. He recalled the "blond giggler" tearing around with the other kids at the party. Before I left, I promised I would do for others what he had done for me. I would listen, believe, and empower those least likely to believe in themselves. I would plant seeds.

The internship year is a book in itself. Everything people say about the rigors and stresses of medical internships is true. That year was the most painful, draining, and grueling period in my life. For a hundred hours a week, or more, I was immersed in labor and delivery, assisting with surgeries, outpatient clinics, internal medicine, and on call for the emergency room. Randy and Sonja were largely on their own.

I was only rarely able to include Sonja in my daily routine. The chief resident and I had daughters about the same age. If our overnight call coincided on weekends, we'd bring our kids to work.

One morning on rounds, a group of us came around the corner to find Sonja and her playmate dressed in oversized scrubs, wearing hospital booties, holding clipboards, and walking in purposeful circles.

"What are you two doing?" one of the attending physicians asked.

"We're making rounds," they announced, as if that was pretty plain to see.

As part of my internship training I observed procedures in the abortion clinic and learned from skilled, caring, and compassionate doctors. One day our chief resident introduced me to a patient and told her I would be doing her abortion. I remember sitting down at the foot of the bed and flashing back to my own awful procedure.

I pushed back from the bed and stood up. I asked the patient to sit so we could talk. She had already received thorough counseling, but we talked more about the procedure, its alternatives, the risks, and possible complications. I wanted to make sure she understood everything and had all her questions answered. I wanted to make sure she was clear in her choice. I was, of course, imagining myself when I had been in need of these very same things.

The procedure went well, though I know I was slow. I did three more procedures that day, learning from each one. With a growing confidence, I saw that I could do this and do it well.

At the end of one year, I left the program, certified as a general practitioner. As quickly as we could, Randy, Sonja, and I packed up to return to the Midwest.

Randy had begun taking courses toward an engineering degree in Portland, and we agreed that he should complete his degree in the Twin Cities. We chose to move to Cambridge, Minnesota, an hour away from Grantsburg, Wisconsin, where much of our family lived. I'd have to commute to the job I'd accepted at the Grantsburg clinic and hospital, but Randy would have a shorter commute to school in St. Paul.

It was the summer of 1988, and I was a bit apprehensive about returning to work in my hometown. I considered it a temporary situation while Randy finished school. There were two full-time physicians in Grantsburg, with a third, Dr. Hartzell, moving into retirement. Dr. Hartzell had been there since 1949; he was a loved and respected fixture in the community.

My first weekend on call was the Annual Water-Skip contest. Grantsburg bears a sign declaring a population of

1,462, but on that weekend it swells with 10,000 spectators and participants for the insane activity of racing snowmobiles across open water. Inevitably, there is too much drinking, too many accidents, and a little hospital emergency room set on overdrive.

Dr. Hartzell lived just up the street and stopped by to see how things were going more than once that weekend. Miraculously, we found time to sit and chat for a few minutes. I remembered him coming to our home when I was six years old and very sick with rheumatic fever. Later, when I took a fall off the neighbor's pony and broke my arm, he set the break and was the first to sign my cast.

He had been our family doctor in the truest sense of the word. Dr. Hartzell had stuck with the community for years when other doctors had come and gone. Finally I was able to bring the conversation around to what I really wanted to discuss: abortion.

Throughout the United States in the years before abortion was legal, there had been a network of clergy connecting women who wanted abortions with doctors they knew were safe. Dr. Hartzell was one of them. He told me that he always believed that these decisions had to be handled between individual women and their doctors.

When women came to him, whether they were referred from out of the area or local women he had known for years, he would schedule the operating room for a "D & C." D stands for dilation, and C stands for curettage. It refers to a method of opening the cervix and cleaning out the uterus. It is usually a therapeutic procedure in response to abnormal uterine bleeding. It can also be a diagnostic procedure to gather uterine lining, looking for dysplasia or cancer.

The patients coming to Dr. Hartzell for D & Cs, however, were pregnant. The procedure would remove the pregnancy early in the first trimester. The word "abortion" would never appear on the chart. No one asked the obvious questions, but he told me that "there were starting to be some rumblings in the community" about it.

We were both concerned about what this would mean for me, as I planned to continue the practice but would now chart it as an abortion. It was, after all, 1988, and abortion had been legal in the United States since 1973. There was no need to hide, and hiding it only contributed to the negative spin some people try to put on it.

The hospital board had other ideas. Under pressure from a few community members, they had a closed meeting to set into effect a policy that forbid all elective abortions at the hospital. I was furious, but my hands were tied. Dr. Hartzell was retiring and not ready to fight this battle with me. I went to the next open board meeting to try to discuss the issue. I was told that "unwanted pregnancies don't happen in this community" by one of the board members. As I looked around the room, I personally knew that abortion had been a choice made by family members of at least two of the people sitting on the board. I kept quiet, but I wondered if they even recognized their hypocrisy. Over and over, I tried to make my case, but they would not budge.

For the next few months I referred patients with unwanted pregnancies to a clinic in St. Paul, a two-hour drive away. Then one day a woman I had known since we were children came to me. She already had two kids, was living on a shoestring budget, had no health insurance, and was pregnant. She and I talked a long time about the options, and she was clear in her decision to have an abortion. She asked me to do it. She was adamant about not going to a doctor she didn't know, and she did not want to travel to St. Paul.

My choices were clear, but none of them were very good. If I sent her away, I was failing as her doctor and as her friend. If I did the abortion openly at the hospital, I would likely get fired. I chose instead to risk my job and my credibility, but it was a choice I made for that patient and for a number of others over the following year. It was a choice mandated by circumstance, much like Dr. Hartzell's decision had been to perform procedures in a clandestine manner. A decision forced by a difficult reality.

I would first discuss the entire approach with the patient. Then I had her come to the clinic after hours. I would insert laminaria into the cervix and send her home, with instructions to come to the emergency room at the hospital the following morning at six AM, when I would be on call. The laminaria would cause the cervix to open a small amount, and bleeding would begin. Basically, it starts a miscarriage. When the patient came to the emergency room the next morning with vaginal bleeding, cramping, and a positive pregnancy test, a therapeutic D & C, using vacuum aspiration, was the treatment of choice. I could take her into the operating room and complete the abortion, never charting the use of the laminaria.

Much as it grated to have to operate in this surreptitious, underground fashion, I was not about to let down women who needed me. And I felt an unexpected connection with Dr. Hartzell and scores of other practitioners throughout the world who had done what they felt was right in circumstances less than ideal.

Time in Grantsburg wasn't all work related. I had many relatives and friends nearby whom I could visit, and I arranged to keep a horse at a friend's stable. Riding had always been my solace in difficult times and an everyday joy whenever I had the opportunity.

When I was on call but nothing was happening at the hospital, I'd escape for a quick ride, not even changing out of my scrubs. Several times an ambulance call came in while I was out riding bareback. The hospital would radio me, and a police squad car would meet me at the trail. One of the officers, a high school friend, would ride the horse back to the stable, while I hopped into the squad car and raced off to meet the ambulance.

Summer passed, and I stayed on in Grantsburg. All along, my mother was my confidant. She was the one I had called after my abortion in Portland. She knew about my training in abortions. I had vented my frustrations to her about the Grantsburg hospital. She was one of the few who knew about my underground activities and who completely understood the phenomenon of community blindness.

The next winter I heard about a march being planned—the March for Women's Lives. When I told Mom about it, she said, "Let's go. Let's all go, even Sonja."

In early April of 1989, we headed for Washington, DC, three generations of women. We arrived two days early and stayed in a single, cheap room twenty minutes from downtown.

We were too nervous to try the subway system at first, so we walked to the march headquarters at the National Organization for Women (NOW) office and volunteered to do whatever we could to help. We stuffed envelopes and made signs and put together clipboards for gathering signatures. Mostly, we talked.

There were women working in that room from every layer and corner of America. Lawyers and store clerks. Factory workers, nurses, the unemployed. Elderly women, young women, mothers, and grandmothers. Women who had hitchhiked across the country. A busload of students from a Catholic college. Hour after hour we talked about our reasons for coming. We shared the life events that had inspired us to action. I felt caught up in the energy of a solidarity I had never before known.

Even though it was cold and drizzling rain on the morning of April 5, solid masses of people kept emerging from the Metro stations, carrying signs, calling out slogans, united in their demands for women's rights. We joined with tens of thousands, all jostling toward the Washington Monument. From there we marched down Pennsylvania Avenue. All the while, the three of us circulated, taking down names of marchers on clipboards, documenting the event. People stretched for miles down the route. The official count was six hundred thousand.

At the end of the march, during the music and speeches, my attention was riveted on a particular speaker, Molly Yard, who was then president of NOW. Everyone has gifts, she was saying. Everyone has some special gift, talent, or energy. All of us can do more than we are doing right now. We all need to be brave, to put ourselves on the line for this cause. We know what it is we can do, and we know how to do it. We just need to start.

For a long time I stood there, thinking. I don't remember the rest of the speech, or any of the others for that matter. Her call to action had sunk in. I knew I had more I could do.

Two weeks after returning home I began making inquiries. I called one of the St. Paul clinics that provided abortions. When I told the director that I was a doctor, that I wanted to help in clinics that provided abortions, and that I was trained in the vacuum aspiration procedure, I don't think she really believed me. Doctors who were trained and willing to work in the clinics were very few and very far between.

Within days I was sitting in a meeting with clinic directors who had traveled to meet me from Fargo, North Dakota, Appleton and Milwaukee, Wisconsin, and Minneapolis and St. Paul, Minnesota. For more than an hour they grilled me with technical questions. They wanted detailed descriptions of procedures, explanations of possible complications and how I would treat them, follow-up concerns, my philosophy. At the end of our meeting they were satisfied I knew what I was talking about.

Then they began explaining the hardships I would face if I decided to begin the work on a regular basis. They told me about the emotional toll, the stresses my family would face, and the difficulties presented by protestors. I heard their words, nodded my head, and reassured them that I was fully aware of all that and I was still prepared to work in their clinics as an abortion provider.

I nodded my head, spoke the words, and told myself I was prepared. I didn't have a clue.

Crimes Committed by Abortion Protesters
in the United States and Canada, 1977–2005:

» 7 murders

» 17 attempted murders

» 52 bombings

» 180 arsons

» 89 invasions

» 1,211 incidents of vandalism

» 1,341 trespasses

» 100 acid attacks

» 655 anthrax threats

» 146 cases of assault and battery

» 375 death threats

» 3 kidnappings

» 96 burglaries

» 480 cases of stalking

One in five clinics experiences blockades, invasions, arsons, bombings, chemical attacks, stalking, gunfire, physical assaults, threats of bombs, death, or arson.

—FEMINIST MAJORITY FOUNDATION

— chapter five

On June 22, 1989, I flew to Milwaukee from Minneapolis, was picked up at the airport by clinic staff, and came to work at one of several clinics owned and operated by Susan Hill's National Women's Health Organization.

I was the only doctor that day, feeling those first-day jitters. I'd done hundreds of abortions, but never as the sole physician in a facility. It felt like the most important and dramatic moment of my professional life. I was utterly focused on the day ahead, my mind full of thoughts, images of patients, the approach I wanted to take as I began establishing my style.

My escort dropped me off and went to park. A group of protesters circled the front door, a dozen or more. When I walked toward them, they assumed I was a patient coming for an abortion.

"Mommy, don't kill your baby. Let us help you. You'll die in there!" they shouted. "You'll bleed to death. You'll never get pregnant again. Mommy, Mommy don't kill me!"

Their shouts barely registered. I was concentrating hard on the work waiting for me. I shouldered through them without breaking stride and found more welcoming staff inside. They showed me where to find the scrubs and where to change my clothes, and gave me a quick tour of the clinic. They were warm and friendly, obviously appreciative, but I am sure more than a little anxious about this new doctor.

I shared that anxious undercurrent. There were fourteen patients on the schedule. Today I would have no supporting doctor to turn to for advice. The responsibility was all mine.

The head nurse welcomed me with a cup of coffee, and we sat down to talk through the patient flow details. I liked what I heard about counseling approaches, established protocols, and patient priorities. Out in the hall I saw one of the clinical assistants gently escorting a patient into a room for an ultrasound. The staff member spoke softly and directly to the patient, obviously treating her with respect and compassion. As I began to negotiate the charts, I felt myself relax. My sense of comfort increased when I actually started seeing patients.

The time passed quickly. I met patient after patient, established a rapport with each one, earned their trust. It felt so good to finally be in a clinic, providing the service I knew was vital to the physical and emotional health of women. Time and again I flashed back to my own abortion. I carried those memories into every meeting. It reinforced my confidence and commitment to hear the concerns women shared. It was even more reassuring to see patients in the recovery room. There the women were comfortable, healthy, and relieved, and in a palpable way they seemed empowered.

It's been nearly twenty years since that first day in Milwaukee, but one woman remains sharp in my memory. She was well dressed, articulate, composed. Every hair was in place. Perfect makeup. When we talked before the abortion, she was straightforward and unemotional. She revealed no inner turmoil and answered my questions briefly, but with obvious determination. I tried to get her to engage with me on a more personal level, but she remained businesslike and direct. No hand wringing or outpouring of emotions.

During the procedure she remained completely still and calm. She showed no sign of fear or anxiety. She made no sound, asked no questions. I talked as I worked, explaining what I was doing and telling her to please speak up if she was uncomfortable.

When the abortion was finished, I rolled back from the bed on my stool and began picking up instruments. When the nurse began checking her blood pressure, the patient lifted her head and caught my eye.

"We're through?" she asked in a hushed voice.

I nodded.

She let her head down again and spoke to the ceiling in a slightly louder voice. "Does this mean I am not pregnant anymore?" There was a new tone in her voice. She sounded like she was ready to explode.

"Yes, it does," I almost whispered back.

"YEEAAAAAAAAYYY! YES! YES! YES!" The shriek of primal relief echoed in the room. I jerked away in surprise, almost tipping backward on my stool.

Her arms shot up in triumph, like an athlete after a game-winning point. I had thought she was immune to emotion. All of this had been carefully pent up—all the tension, the weight of her situation, all of it locked behind her impeccable facade. Until now.

Now she wore a smile that wouldn't fade. She released a flood of concerns she was free of, some of them planted by the words of the protesters out front. She and I talked about the insensitive actions and outright lies spewed by the protesters. We talked about how hard it had been for her to walk through their gauntlet, and how difficult it would be for women who weren't as strong as she was. Young women, for instance. Women with no one to turn to for support, women who didn't know the facts about abortion.

Later that first day, when I left the clinic, I saw the protesters differently. They were no longer just a nuisance. They were a force that had a negative impact on my patients, planting unnecessary fear and guilt in women at this vulnerable crossroads, as they weighed whether to end an unwanted pregnancy. Their rhetoric and self-righteous pleading were misleading and alarming. I knew, looking at them, that the last thing they cared about was the safety and well-being of the women I had seen that day.

Within a month I added another clinic, flying to Appleton, Wisconsin, to work for Maggie Cage, a woman full of commitment and understanding who was also a tough, battle-hardened warrior. I used all my vacation days, my usual day off, and all my Saturdays to provide abortions in Appleton and Milwaukee. The atmosphere and attitudes of the staff were exactly what I had been hoping for.

My contract as a general practitioner in Grantsburg was up for renewal in October. I had been there just fifteen months. I relished the joy of delivering babies for women I'd grown up with and taking care of friends and relatives in the emergency room, the clinic, or the nursing home. But it often cut too close to the bone. Every time one of the elders died, part of me died with them. Taking care of chronically sick people who had abused their bodies for decades did not bring me much satisfaction.

Juxtaposed against the new energy I felt, and the sense of performing meaningful work on behalf of women, there was no contest. I did not renew my contract. Instead I offered my skills as an abortion provider to three additional clinics, one in Fargo, North Dakota, one in Duluth, Minnesota, and one in St. Paul.

These clinics were owned or managed by women who understood that no one should be turned away because of financial constraints. They understood that patients needed clear, accurate information and care that was emotionally supportive as well as physically safe.

Susan Hill owned the clinic in Fargo as well as the one in Milwaukee. I started traveling there regularly. In Duluth the clinic was run by a strong, feminist woman with a great staff. The clinic in St. Paul was part of a large nonprofit organization. The manager was my main point of contact, and she was as dedicated and kind as anyone I've ever worked with. She was an excellent liaison between the umbrella administration and the clinic staff, and put patient care issues first.

As the weeks passed, what grew more powerful in me was the fundamental commitment to patients and to the cause of keeping reproductive rights safe and legal. I was free of the conservative, oppressive bosses who lived in denial and demanded allegiance to the financial bottom line over full treatment. Free of edicts to spend no more than ten minutes with a teenager experiencing her first pelvic exam and wanting birth control advice.

"Give them a Pap, hand them birth control pills, and move on," I'd been instructed in Grantsburg. Now I was free of off-site administrators with no community knowledge telling me to stop seeing "welfare patients" because they didn't bring in any money. More to the point, I was finally free of secretive, furtive abortions.

Work was invigorating and gratifying, but there was a price to pay. My schedule was exhausting. And it played havoc with my family life. I felt as if I were constantly in a state of jet lag, rotating between airports and clinics and vehicles.

"Sue," Randy said one weekend. "It's your mom's birthday next week. Let's find a day to go see your folks. Your dad isn't doing so well, and Sonja always loves seeing them."

"I know," I said, "but tomorrow I fly to Appleton and don't get back until late Tuesday. Wednesday I drive to Duluth and won't be home until late."

"What about Thursday night?" he asked.

"Nope. I go to Milwaukee this week, so I fly out Thursday morning and don't get back until Friday night, and I've agreed to work on Saturday in St. Paul."

"Sunday?"

"Please, I need one day at home," I said. "You and Sonja go if you want, but I have to have one day staying put."

If Randy was disappointed, he hid it well. He was totally supportive of my work and the choices I'd made, but I know there were many times he had to swallow hard and walk away. Sonja had her own busy schedule, full of swim team practices and homework and friends, but she missed the trips to see family.

My professional life was hitting sonic speed, heady and rewarding, but I was suffering from tunnel vision.

Part of my work preoccupation came from the fact that I still had so much to learn. One of the counselors in Appleton was a clinic veteran named Dottie. She taught me valuable lessons about how to talk with patients and how to really hear what they are saying. Dottie always made it clear that we did abortions for the woman, not for her partner or husband or mother. For the woman. It was her choice, and she needed to completely own that. Dottie taught me that no matter how good the counseling was before the abortion, there would be times when issues wouldn't come to the surface until the woman was actually undressed and facing the beginning of the procedure. I learned to ask every patient if she was absolutely sure of her decision.

"Is anyone pushing you or telling you that you have to do this?" I'd ask.

Any hesitation whatsoever and I stopped and asked her to get dressed again, and we talked more. It wasn't uncommon for me to send her away to reconsider her options. My biggest fear has always been to do an abortion on someone who will later come to regret it.

In the early years, when issues of this nature came up, the staff and administration always allowed the time and resources to support a woman's choice and to help her reach a point of resolution. The patient took first priority. That supportive, nurturing environment within the clinic made it possible for me to endure the increasing efforts of the anti-abortion zealots and to overcome the hate they directed at me.

By the summer of 1990 the protestors had figured out that I was one of the doctors. When I approached a clinic entrance, tried to get out of an airport, or walked from my car to a clinic entrance, they went into a frenzy.

"Murderer!" they screamed. "Baby killer!"

I dreaded seeing them—every time. How could they hold up a Bible while screaming through clenched teeth? When in a public place and being singled out, I cringed at the looks people gave me. I hated the thought that anyone witnessing this spectacle would believe I actually *did* kill babies. My stomach would knot and churn.

Sometimes I was close enough to see the hateful, twisted facial expressions of the protesters. It was horrifying. Their voices were shrill and loud and unstoppable. I was engulfed in a tornado of frenzied emotion, out of control and very dangerous. I fought the urge to panic, to flee, but I never reacted outwardly, never responded to their taunts, never made eye contact. When they tried to block my way, I'd shove past, hurry on.

"Baby killer! Their blood is on your hands, Susan!"

Entering a clinic, I would often stop to look back and see how the patients were faring. Many times clinic escorts were available to help the patients get through the protesters, but not always. Without the escorts present, and sometimes even when they were, protesters would rush at a patient on the sidewalk, surrounding her and shouting awful rhetoric. They reminded me of a pack of wolves. You could see their frustration when a woman refused to stop and talk to them, but pushed her way into the clinic instead.

The protestors became more and more organized and sophisticated. They got better at deciphering my helter-skelter schedule, knew when to expect me at various clinics, called ahead to their collaborators when I left one airport for another. They followed me in cars and communicated by walkie-talkie and cell phone. I felt as if I were in a spy movie, always watching my rearview mirror, looking for the enemy's face in the crowds.

Sometimes I'd leave in the dead of night and drive five hours rather than face the airport scene. I never checked baggage. The thought of waiting at a baggage turnstile surrounded by antis was too much.

At this point, my schedule required daily flights or drives of two hundred miles or more. At least three nights a week I was in a motel room. Most weeks, Sunday was my only day off. Trying to stay one step ahead of the protesters became a game of nerves.

Within a year of my first visit to the Milwaukee clinic, the protesters were no longer simply circling the entrance and shouting their insults. They had taken to physical blockades, locking themselves together and forming a human barrier. I routinely had to wait outside the building for the police to come, wait while they methodically arrested and removed each person so I could get into the door. It was either that or break through myself—*physically* break through.

Some days the antis were sitting on the ground blocking the door, and the clinic staff would push them out of the way by forcing the door open. I would climb over their bodies, actually step right on these people, to get in.

In several towns, the protesters who were arrested suffered no consequences. The Milwaukee city attorney refused to prosecute them, for example, which meant that they'd have a brief ride down to the police station, be released within minutes, and be back in front of the clinic later the same day. Some were arrested more than a hundred times in one year and never served time or paid a fine.

It became necessary to vary my routine and even the means by which I came and went from the clinic in Milwaukee. There was a back door to the clinic, rarely used because of the poorly maintained alley. I was given the key, however, and on occasion would enter through it. I typically arrived in a taxi from the airport and would let staff know my approximate arrival time. They would try to watch for me.

I had also begun writing in a journal on a regular basis in order to process some of the insanity. I would write on airplanes, in motel rooms, in the clinics while waiting for the day to begin, and at home sitting up late at night, when images and stories filled my head, preventing the sleep I was so in need of.

Journal Entry, August 1990:

Scared. So scared.
　　Hard to write.
　　Hard to think.
　　Heart pounding.
　　Tried to avoid protesters in front. Hid in back seat of taxi. Went to back door 10 minutes ago. Two men there. Had just gotten out of cab, keys in one hand and mobile phone in other. Phone set to call front desk. Routine safety measure. Thank God.

One man grabbed me and slammed me up against a parked van. His face in my face. Screaming at me.

"YOU KILLER! YOU KILLER!"

"YOU DESERVE TO DIE."

"STOP KILLING BABIES, SUSAN!"

I struggled. Fought to get free. Would get away from the van by just inches and they would throw me against it. Over and over. Screaming. All three of us. Almost slow motion. I hit SEND on the phone and hoped someone would hear me and figure it out. Felt like no one would ever come. Kept trying to pull away. Lost my voice. Tried and tried but couldn't scream again. Felt my hips slam into the side of the van again. Heard another voice. Back door was open! Attackers briefly let me go and I ran for it. Staff member grabbed my arm and tried to pull me in. Attacker on other arm. Tug-of-war. Is this really happening? Able to scream again.

Finally got pulled into a heap on the floor just inside the door. Men took off running. Feel like I'm still sitting in a frantic dream. Nightmare. Trying to settle down. Need to gather myself enough to see patients. Need to cry. Can't stop shaking.

The protesters became enough of a danger and daily hassle that friends and staff suggested I consider using disguises. It seemed like a possible solution, and at least a way of avoiding some of the direct confrontations. I began collecting clothes and hats and scarves completely out of character for me. I practiced making myself up and tried to change my mannerisms like an actress assuming different characters.

Journal Entry, January 27, 1991:

Snowstorm. Just dropped Martha off at the airport here in Fargo. Right now feel like I'm in another world. Bought a wig last night in Duluth. Martha and I knew it was serious stuff, but couldn't stop giggling. Hair salon salesperson thought we were nuts and showed obvious surprise when I bought a good quality wig.

Conversation at one point as I tried on an auburn, curly haired wig, shoulder length:

Clerk: "That really doesn't look much like you."

Me: "Good. That is the idea."

Clerk to Martha: "Well, she really does look good with hair."

Martha and I doubled up in laughter. Martha leaning against the wall, tears running down her face. I was sitting on the stool with this long, curly hair over my half-inch-long, straight, gray hair, laughing so hard I was snorting. "Sold," I half cried. "Got any red lipstick to clash?" But by now I was feeling a terror in my stomach. My tears were out of real fear, not humor.

We left and headed for Fargo. 5 hour drive in good weather. Took us 7 in a blizzard. Sometimes down to 20 mph. So tired.

Then I donned my wig, put on my new make-up and black stretch pants, red shoes, a red polyester blouse and plaid blazer. Drove Martha to the airport dressed like that. Our good-byes are usually teary and so sad. This time we giggled. Why? Because of my ridiculous outfit. And to hide our fear.

I got to the clinic with no staff knowing about the new me. Had prearranged with Jane to have a name on the appointment list so I'd be let in and treated like a patient. Went up the stairs to admitting as instructed, excused myself to the restroom, changed clothes, washed my face and shoved the wig through the pass-door into the lab where urine samples usually go. Freaked out Carol in lab. Explained to staff later and they were OK with it all. Protesters hadn't a clue when I had come in. That was the only good part. It feels so awful. Why do I have to do this to go to work? WHY? Just to avoid taunts or the threat of having the car I'm in stopped by some screaming fanatics? I can't stand it when they get so close to me. There is so much hate in their eyes.

People said how smart I must feel to have fooled the protesters. I just feel drained.

I made friends with a man who often flew on the same commuter flight as I did to Appleton every Tuesday. Sometimes we sat together, but our conversations always centered on his life, his work, his family, not on mine. I would always hang back when we got to Appleton, taking extra time to gather my things so I would be the last one off the plane and the other passengers wouldn't see the circus created by the protesters when I entered the airport.

I sat near him one of the first times I wore a disguise. It was a hideous costume—brightly beaded jean jacket, an auburn wig, polyester pants, and a big purse. I hated the deceit, the fact that I was going to these extremes to avoid the harassment. And now it meant I couldn't sit and have a pleasant conversation with a friend.

He didn't recognize me, and at the airport in Appleton I walked out with all the other passengers. The protesters never suspected. I walked right past as they craned their necks, searching the small group of passengers. That anonymity was the only thing that made the demeaning effort worth it.

A day later, on the return flight, I sat across the narrow aisle from my friend, undisguised. I had the unmistakable jean jacket folded carefully in my lap so that only the denim showed. We talked as usual, but at one point I dropped something and in bending over, the jacket fell open into the aisle. His eyes moved to the gaudy coat, back to my face.

"That was you," he said finally. "That was you yesterday. What the hell is going on? Who are you, anyway? What's the gig? Are you running drugs or something?" He was really angry with me.

I didn't want to explain. The airplane was my place of refuge and anonymity. What would he think? But he kept interrogating me, unrelenting.

"No, no, it's nothing like drugs. It's much simpler. No. It's much more complicated. I'm a doctor. I do abortions. Every week I fly here to work in a clinic. There are people who try to stop me from doing my work. People who harass me. Haven't you ever seen the protesters at the airport? They are waiting for me. I have had to resort to disguises because I can't stand them in my face anymore."

It all came out at once, in one big gushing confession. We talked the rest of the flight. I told him about my work, my ridiculous schedule, how I got started, the people at the clinics, the confrontations that had become such a torment.

After that, whenever we flew together, he waited for me as we got off the plane; with his arm wrapped tightly around my shoulders, we barreled through the protesters together. He made sure I was safely in a taxi before heading his own way.

For the first time I understood that I had potential allies as well as enemies.

I continued to use whatever means I had to get into the clinics. Disguises, riding in the trunk of a car, sometimes arriving at five in the morning and sleeping in the clinic until the rest of the staff arrived. It was exhausting and frustrating. It felt as if I were letting the protesters dictate the rules of interaction, as if I had stooped to lies and subterfuge. I didn't want to interact on their terms, sink to their level.

It was the patients who kept me going. Their situations, their needs, their genuine thanks and relief. Without knowing it, they were the ones doing the comforting. They were helping me through situations I could never have imagined.

On the weeks that I drove the 240 miles to Fargo I would stop on the edge of town and call the clinic for a "protester-of-the-day" report. When I called one day, the activity was particularly bad. The clinic director didn't hesitate in expressing her concern.

"They're stopping every car," Jane told me. "If anyone inside looks like you or a patient, they chain themselves to the axle or lie in front of the vehicle."

I knew the scene only too well. Protesters jumping on cars or lying in the road while someone wormed underneath and locked on to the axle with a bicycle lock or chain. Any open window in the car would have anti-abortion propaganda shoved through it. Flyers would be slapped on car windshields. Frightened occupants would be extremely upset.

"I'm sending two volunteers out in a car to meet you at the mall parking lot," Jane instructed. "You can hide in the back or under blankets. Just stay in the car if they stop it."

By the time the volunteers drove up, I'd put on a blond wig and a heavy coat of makeup. I wore a long black jumper, tennis shoes, and sunglasses. My escorts turned in open-mouthed surprise when I approached them and spoke.

"It's Dr. Wicklund!" one of them exclaimed. "I can't believe it!"

"I want you to take me to the McDonald's and drop me off. I don't want to be seen with anyone they'll recognize. I'm walking the last two blocks alone."

They didn't like my idea at all, but I was adamant. I knew they were worried about going back to the clinic without me and explaining to Jane. I made sure they would tell the main guard in the front of the clinic to watch for me and let me in when I caught his eye.

On my own, without the protection of a car or friends, I walked toward the clinic, all the while fearing that my true identity would be discovered. What would happen if these people actually got their hands on me? I could see the crowd gathered there, one hundred of them, I guessed, maybe more. All people who hated me, whose only objective was to keep me from my work. Under the pious, prayerful guise of religion, they were after control: Control of me. Control of the women coming to the clinic for help. Control of anyone who believed differently than they.

I had to act as if I belonged. At the edge of the crowd I began mingling, trying to fit with their body language, trying to put myself completely into the act. Being among them, brushing shoulders, and hearing their hateful, vicious lies were almost too much.

"Who is that in that car?" one would yell as the next vehicle approached the parking lot. "Stop that car!" The crowd surged toward the target, and I moved right along with them. I heard myself shouting their awful words just to play the part. Slowly I moved with the human waves, closer and closer to the building.

The nearer I got to the front the more frightening it became. How long could I keep it up? Was it the cumulative effect of being in their midst that was taking my breath away? There was sweat running down my face and my back. I knew I had to stay calm and keep acting as if I belonged. They were shouting, frenzied, on the fringe of sanity. Surrounded by them, choked by their energy, I felt claustrophobic, almost physically sick. They knew I was scheduled to arrive at the clinic soon. Any car could be carrying me.

I gained the front sidewalk. All the crowd pressure was at my back. This terrible, righteous, oblivious hatred beat against me, pounded against the building that offered me safety. So close.

Finally, I was at the front lines. I took off my sunglasses as I moved closer to the guard. He was looking right past me. I was right in his face, silently shouting with my eyes, "It's me! It's me!" He kept looking around me, over me, searching the crowd. Then his eyes found mine, stopped. Color drained from his face. I nodded. He lifted his outstretched arm and moved slightly to the side, opening up a path that I darted through.

Five steps from one world to another. I gulped in a huge breath. I had been holding my breath for a long time. It was all I could do to stumble up the steps and pound on the door. A staff person recognized me and threw open the door. I never looked back, couldn't face the vision of what I'd come through.

Once inside I couldn't go any further. I tore the wig off and collapsed on a flight of stairs. Great, whooping sobs racked my body. Makeup ran in streaks down my face. All the bravado and fortitude I'd summoned to protect myself deserted me, turning to unbelievable relief and fatigue. And I couldn't stop crying.

Never again. Never again, I kept thinking.

A woman came down the stairs and sat next to me. She had no idea who I was, what I'd been through, but she put her arm around me and rocked, holding me like a child as I sobbed. We sat together, strangers consoling one another.

Two hours later that same woman was on the operating table, one of my patients, and it was my turn to help her through her ordeal. I was struck again with the affirmation that people are by and large good. I realized how important it is to trust that the good energy and kindness you put out will always find its way back to you.

Never again, I kept repeating to myself during the day. Never will I wear disguises again. Never will I hide and sneak around at crazy hours. I will not stoop to their level, play their game. I can't live with that any longer.

The protesters had been paying attention, however. They interpreted my behavior as a statement of vulnerability and shame. They thought that I would go to any lengths to avoid confrontation. They also discovered that I was a mother with a teenage daughter, a vulnerability they might exploit.

On the morning of October 3, 1991, I woke to the sound of people shouting, "Susan kills babies!" outside our bedroom window. "Susan kills babies!" I heard again. Must be a nightmare, I thought. I'm home. I am not at work. I am in my bed, right next to Randy. But I was awake. I was in my own bed. This was real. A cold nausea swept through me. Nausea and gut-level fear.

We, the remnant of God-fearing men
and women of the United States of Amerika,
do officially declare war on the entire
child killing industry. . . . Our Most Dread
Sovereign Lord God requires that
whosoever sheds man's blood, by man
shall his blood be shed.

—EXCERPT FROM MANUAL PUBLISHED BY
THE ARMY OF GOD, AN UNDERGROUND
NETWORK OF DOMESTIC TERRORISTS
DEDICATED TO USING VIOLENCE AS A MEANS
TO END THE PRACTICE OF LEGAL ABORTION

— chapter six

I woke Randy and stopped him from turning on the lamp. He sensed the urgency in my voice and groggily began to take in the scene outside.

"Call the police. I'm going to check on Sonja," I choked out in a whisper.

Terror hammered in my throat. I flew down the stairs to Sonja's basement bedroom. In those slow-motion ten seconds, horrible scenarios rushed through my head. But she was sleeping soundly, completely oblivious to the obscenity outside. I kissed her, touched her warm face, and backed thankfully out of her room.

Randy met me on the stairs. "Police are on their way," he said. We started to prowl around the house, avoiding windows. No curtains anywhere, I realized. There had never been any need for them. Our house sat in six acres of woods at the end of a driveway that itself was at the end of a three-mile dead-end road. That isolation had always been a comfort. Curtains and drapes had never occurred to me.

I found the only place without any windows at all. The shower. I sat down in the stall, hugging my knees to my chest, trying to swallow the anger and fear, fighting as hard as I could to hold on to some control.

Just the week before, our nearby town had been leafleted by the anti-abortion fanatics. They had put up "wanted" posters all over town—on cars, on bulletin boards for public announcements, even on the school grounds. There was a picture of my face with the words "Wanted for the Murder of Children." It had caused quite a stir and a rash of letters to the editor in the local paper, most of them condemning the horrendous tactics. For the past week I had avoided going to town, afraid of people's reactions.

The eastern sky was just beginning to lighten, and we could see shadowy figures in the yard and driveway. When headlights approached from down the road, the shapes began to move from our private land. The police cruiser came right up to the house, and when the officer came up the steps, we turned on lights for the first time, opened the door. There, on the porch, the protesters had left a white bassinet with a doll inside. The doll was wrapped in a crocheted afghan and splattered with red paint. Play money had been scattered around.

The officer was our neighbor. We all stood there looking at the garish doll, then went inside.

"How is Sonja going to get to school? I have to get to the airport. Can they do this?" I began pacing back and forth across the kitchen, seething inside. I felt an intense need to escape and outrage that this could be happening. I was used to clinic protesters, but here they were, at my house!

"These people can do this?" I kept asking. The officer seemed as much at a loss as we did. He and Randy discussed options, but I tuned them out. There was nothing reasonable about any of this. The officer eventually used our phone to call for backup. I put on coffee, comforted by that element of routine, and we sat together feeling trapped in our own kitchen.

More police cars arrived. Sonja came upstairs and got ready for school. She kept glancing to me for signals, reading my reactions. I did my best to appear calm and to convince her that everything was under control.

I toasted bagels. "Sit down and eat, Sonja. I'll braid your hair."

"Are you going to work, Mom?" she asked.

"Of course I'm going," I said. "But first we're getting you off to school."

"How?"

"The police will escort you," Randy interjected.

I tried to downplay the people at the end of the driveway. Then I felt an absolute desolation, a complete disconnect from everything I had ever known, while I watched Sonja's head diminish down the driveway in the back window of a police car.

I cringed when the cruiser crept past a banner that read "Susan Kills Babies." I could hear the shouts of the protesters aimed at my daughter. At the end of the drive several dozen antis, men and women ranging in age from twenty to sixty, videotaped Sonja's departure while she hid her face behind a Spanish textbook.

I didn't have to leave for several hours, but once Sonja had gone, I couldn't restrain my need to escape. Randy volunteered to stay home for the day to watch the house.

"It's okay," he insisted, "you need to get to work. You have patients."

"But what about your classes?" I asked.

"I can make the work up next week. Your patients can't wait."

We looked at each other for a long moment. I thought of all the ways he had sacrificed his needs and comfort for my career. His eyes held mine. I saw that he was just as appalled and just as determined as I felt.

"Okay," I said, taking his hand and holding tight.

Two police cars escorted me down the drive after we pulled a white sheet off my car that was spray-painted with "No More Dead Babies." At the end we confronted a mass of protesters. They parted just enough to allow the cars out, like guards at a military checkpoint, as if they were in charge, as if they controlled who came and went. In the days and weeks to follow, it became obvious that to a great extent they could, in fact, control much of our lives.

I eventually made my way to the Minneapolis airport, flew to Milwaukee, and put in two full days of work. I don't remember the patients, the routine protesters, what the weather was like, what I wore. I remember only the preoccupation with my home and my family, the anxiety and uncertainty. How could they do this? How could they violate my home, disrupt our lives so rudely? Did the police have them out yet? How long would it last?

A dozen times each day I called home. The antis had leafleted my town again with flyers full of the usual hyperbole. "Your neighbor, Susan Wicklund, is a terrorist to the unborn. Every day she tears helpless, defenseless babies from their mother's wombs, tears their bodies apart. . . ."

I called Mom from work and filled her in.

"Are you all okay?" she asked.

"Yes, we're fine. Sonja got to school, and Randy stayed home."

"Don't worry, honey," she said. "I'll come over soon and help out. I don't think I'll tell your dad everything yet, but don't worry. We can get past this."

Randy stayed home a second day out of fear for our property. Little did we know that this would continue for weeks and that he would be forced to drop out of a semester of college. I tried unsuccessfully to block the insistent distractions from my mind while I worked. I used the unflappable calm of Mom's words to steel my determination.

On my return to the Minneapolis airport I was completely caught up in my thoughts, anxious to see that Sonja and Randy were safe. I abandoned my usual vigilance, wondering instead how Sonja had come home from school that afternoon, whether the antis would be waiting for me at the end of my driveway.

The elevator opened on the fifth floor of the parking garage. It struck me how empty and devoid of people it was at ten P.M. I began walking toward my car, listening to the sound of my own footsteps. I saw movement inside a van about fifty feet away. Three people emerged, two men and a woman, and they all moved purposefully in my direction. Protesters. I knew it with certainty and with a dread that filled me like ice water.

I slowed. My first instinct was to turn and flee, to give in to the panic clawing at my insides. But I had to keep on. I couldn't allow them that triumph, couldn't let the fear take over. They came at me with that infuriating righteousness, that blind indignation that ignored courtesy, discretion, even law—right at me until they stood an arm's length away. I avoided eye contact, looked at their chests, their shoes. I felt like prey.

They began with their stream of words. The words that, by then, were stamped in my mind, words fueled with venom: "Susan, you have to stop killing babies. Susan, you are a killer of the unborn. Your victims have no say." My name in their mouths was always the most repugnant sound. How dare they speak my name as if they knew me. Their words ran together in a meaningless babble.

My body felt hot, as if my skin couldn't contain the heat building inside. I knew exactly how vulnerable I was, how outnumbered, how completely ambushed I was here. I recognized two of them, protesters I'd seen regularly in Appleton, Wisconsin. One of them was a large, violent-looking man. They've come three hundred miles to meet me in a dark parking lot? Are these people crazy?

I couldn't allow them to corner me. I have to make myself big, I thought. Have to be strong and fierce. Overpowering. Can't give in to feeling trapped, to the bone-deep panic. Inside it was as if I were exploding, this heat welling up in a volcanic, explosive rush. For the first time I looked into their faces, two feet away.

"How dare you?!" I screamed. "How dare you?" Over and over the words came. The only words in my mind. Screaming at them. Now I was attacking, stabbing them with my eyes, speeding up, rushing at them. "How DARE you?"

Never before had I even considered speaking to them. "HOW DARE YOU? You go to my home? You terrorize my daughter? You walk all over my land? You self-righteous, lying hypocrites! HOW DARE YOU?" Words were my only weapon, my only power, my bigness. Words and the heated force pushing them out of my body, making my body huge. HUGE!

They stopped. Backed up. I could see shock and indecision register. They exchanged uncertain glances. Now they wouldn't meet my eyes. I kept pushing on them, not letting up, screaming out my rage. Whenever I paused, they started their litany of damnation again, their blind catechism, but the words had lost their power. I shouted them down and pressed onward with my HUGE presence.

Suddenly I was at my car. I unlocked the door and threw my pack inside, started to get in as I watched them over my shoulder. The attackers turned and moved toward their van. Something inside me fired, and I knew I couldn't let them off that easily. I reached into my backpack and grabbed the camera.

"HEY! I'm not done with you! I want your pictures!" I raised my arm high, then swung it forcefully downward, jabbing my finger toward the ground. "Come back here. All of you. I'm not finished!" Between words I could feel my heart racing, this rage barely containable, my body barely capable of coping. "STOP! STOP AND LOOK AT ME!"

They had retreated to their van, clustered together in a confused clump. They hid their faces from me. I ran toward them, began taking pictures, the flash stabbing out again and again in the half-lit space. "Why are you hiding?" I screamed. "You're so proud of what you do, right? Then look at me! LOOK AT ME, YOU COWARD!" The big man turned away, hunched over. "Show your face!! If you are so damn proud, SHOW YOUR FACE!"

I marched back to my car, beginning to shake all over. Got to stay together. Hold it together. Inside. Lock the doors. Start up. The engine revved loudly, a noise big and powerful. Then I squealed back, straight toward the van, stopped just short of it. My heart beat like a charging horse. All the way down the spiraling ramp I laid on the horn, five floors down, loud and furious.

Then the toll booth. Had to find money, act normally, make an exchange. Finally out in the big night, the cool air, and all the heat in me collapsed, all the torrent of emotion fell off. I managed to get on the freeway, shaking fiercely. Got to stay together. My body was still functioning, but the bigness that had empowered me dissolved.

First exit. Can't drive. Can't do anything. Pulled over, actually up onto the sidewalk, stumbled out. I was crying. I sat against the fire hydrant and cried uncontrollably while people passed by. Then I started to vomit, heaving up the terrible fear inside, everything collapsing, sobbing, letting it drain away. The inner screaming subsided, my heart slowed. Periodically I retched, bringing up nothing. Inside, taking the place of heat and fear, I added another layer to my resolve.

For weeks the siege continued. Sonja stayed with her father, David, on weekends whenever possible. David was now living in St. Paul and had remarried, but he saw Sonja regularly. The police car was her school bus many times. My mother would come to stay at the house on days when neither Randy nor I would be there. Protesters stayed outside the house day and night. They would always move aside to let me drive in, but would frequently delay or block me from leaving.

Sometimes they would block me with their bodies; other times they'd haul in huge cement-filled barrels with trucks. Over and over they spread their leaflets around town, six miles away. They called themselves the Lambs of Christ.

Not long before the onslaught, we had signed papers to buy an old farmstead four miles away. We were trying to sell the house we were in, but had not let the real estate agents put up "for sale" signs. Somehow, however, the antis found out. One of the members of the Lambs of Christ masqueraded as a potential buyer. She toured every room, looking at pictures of family members, checking entrances and exits, learning the layout of the house, even finding names of relatives.

Days later I recognized our "potential buyer" as she was being arrested outside the clinic in Fargo, North Dakota.

I often stayed alone at friends' homes so I could be sure of getting to work in the mornings. I took a different route to and from the airport each time, sometimes driving for hours, feeling hunted, watching the cars behind me. Every time I went to my car I checked the tires, looked for nails on the ground. Each time I turned the key I waited for the bomb explosion, held my breath while the engine caught.

The protesters became more and more bold and self-righteous. At every airport I had to run their gauntlet. Life had turned into an awful game. I couldn't trust people, had to suspect every unfamiliar vehicle, every strange voice on the phone. Although I didn't know it then, Shelly Shannon, the woman who years later would shoot Dr. Tiller in Kansas, was a regular at the airport and outside my home with the other Lambs of Christ.

Journal Entry, October 16, 1991:

Slept last night at Kathy's. Arrived at 1:30 am after 6-hour drive from Appleton. Too many antis at the house, so Randy sent Sonja to Kathy's and said I should go there too. Am so frustrated. So sad. So tired. Is this worth it? Am I just being a martyr?

Pulled into the yard. Turned off the car and sat there. Numb. Strange buildings. Not home. But Sonja inside and I needed her comfort as much as she needed mine. Found my way into the house and greeted by Kathy's mom. Talked a bit. Thanked her. Followed her to where Sonja was sleeping.

Stripped down to t-shirt and crawled into bed. Held her. Held her and cried hot tears. No sobbing. No sound. Just rivers of tears.

My God, she is fourteen years old. Fourteen years old and riding to school in police cars. Fourteen years old and sleeping at strange homes because her own home isn't safe or peaceful. Fourteen years old and brave. Am I asking too much of her? Should I send her to live with her Dad? Should I quit? Will she hate me for all this when she is thirty?

Yesterday I felt anger and determination and strength. Today I feel sad and scared and confused. Had to pull my arms away from Sonja at 5:15, shower and dress and head for the airport. The tears haven't stopped.

More than three weeks into this nightmare, Randy, Sonja, and I were at the house on a Wednesday night. I was due in Fargo the next morning for clinic at 9:00 A.M. The three of us only wanted a quiet family evening before I left again. Just one night to have supper together and gather our thoughts.

A great many protesters began collecting outside. We saw a motor home pull up at the end of the drive and then groups of men moving huge cement barrels into place to block our way out. This can't happen, I told myself. I called the police and pleaded with them to come and help. I was told that it was too dangerous for the officers to come in the dark and try to remove the barrels or make arrests. The fifty or sixty protesters far outnumbered the few officers in our entire county.

If the "problem" was still there in the morning, backup help from other counties would be called, and they would start to clear the way once it was light. They said the process could take three to four hours. It meant I wouldn't get out in time to make the four-hour drive to Fargo.

Prisoners in our own home! What if there was a fire or if one of us needed emergency medical help? These people were allowed to break the law and hold us hostage because it was dark outside and they outnumbered the police!

I began pacing around the house. I will not let this happen, I repeated over and over. I had fifteen patients scheduled for the next day, and I was determined to get there. Many of those patients would be traveling four to six hours themselves, missing work or school to go to the appointment, having to arrange child care or a ride or deal with any number of other obstacles. Besides, missing clinic would be a major victory for the protesters. That was not an option.

I made a phone call to a woman in town who had given me her home number and offered help. This would be an extraordinary request, and I woke her up to ask for it, but she agreed.

For the protesters' benefit we played out our normal nightly routine. I didn't tell Sonja anything, but saw her to bed as usual, holding her much longer than normal to say good night, fighting back the lump in my throat. I prepared the coffee pot for the morning. Randy and I brushed our teeth and had lights out by 9:30.

We were lying on top of the bed covers, talking quietly about the details of my plan. I'd be on foot and would meet my friend at a set point on a nearby town road. She'd drive me to our pickup truck, which was parked at a nearby stable where we boarded a few horses. Once I got to the truck, I would drive through the night to Fargo, perhaps catching some sleep at a rest area.

After talking through the details one more time, we lay quietly in the dark. Throughout all of this Randy had been unwaveringly steadfast, completely supportive. He never questioned my commitment, never even hinted that I should quit my work. But I felt the rush of his anxiety when I asked him to get the pistol out of the drawer.

In a lifetime around guns I had never carried one for self-defense. I had never even loaded a gun inside a house before. But I loaded this one.

For a brief moment as I was leaving the bedroom I wondered how crazy I must be, how insane my life had become. But my momentum carried me out the bedroom door and down the stairs to the back door, ready to step out into the night.

Randy had followed me. He stopped me and quietly wrapped his arms around me. We held each other fiercely, silently.

"Call me when you get to Fargo," he whispered.

I stepped back, slung my clothes bag over one shoulder, and held the loaded pistol in both hands.

As soon as I was out the door, I listened intently for strange noises. Noises that didn't belong in a backyard and woods at night. I grew up in the country. Night sounds are generally comforting to me, and those were all I wanted to hear. Nothing more.

Once my eyes had adjusted to the dark and the roar of my heartbeat had quieted, I took two tentative steps away from the side of the house. I had my route planned exactly—down hill on a very narrow, brushy trail that I knew well, down to the edge of a swamp, then along the river on the old trail until I came to the dirt road. There was a turnaround where I'd wait in the ditch for my ride.

The plan was great in theory, but my legs were weak with fear. I wasn't sure I could get beyond those first two steps. Why was I doing this? For the patients? For the principle? To prove something? I went through all the things I'd thought about earlier and came to the same conclusion: I absolutely couldn't let the antis have the victory of keeping me from clinic for even one day. A victory for them would fuel their flames, and they'd increase the pressure even more. I had to keep one step ahead, even when it meant resorting to the sort of tactics I'd never wanted to use again.

I knew the woods well and finally felt ready to head down the hill. I heard voices around the front of the house and saw a cigarette glow about thirty yards off the trail. Every few careful steps I stopped again, thinking of the things Dad taught me about stalking game and about being nearly silent in the woods.

It seemed an eternity. Step by step I made my way, pistol ready, heart louder than my carefully placed footsteps, slowly passing familiar ditches and other landmarks. Please. Please let me make it to the dirt road.

Just as I reached the prearranged spot, a small red car pulled around the corner, came to a smooth stop, and went silent as the engine was cut. "Sue?" I heard the whisper.

"Yes," I breathed, "I'm here." I stuck my head up from the cover of the ditch, shivering with adrenaline.

She delivered me safely to the stables. I walked inside. It was quiet, but full of the sounds and smells of horses. I opened the stall of my black mare, Beauty, and stepped in-side. She roused and turned her head toward me. I buried my face in her neck, breathed in her scent, promised her a long ride on my next free day.

Once in the truck and on my way the questions started pounding in my head again. What's happening? I kept asking myself. I'm not a criminal. I'm not a fugitive. I am sneaking through the woods with a gun in order to get to work. I flashed on a memory: the day in June 1989 when the clinic directors tried to warn me that life could prove to be a real challenge as an abortion provider.

After two hours of driving my adrenaline had been spent, and I could hardly stay awake, yet I knew I wouldn't be able to sleep. I felt a desperate need for a shower and found a motel room at two AM. I stood under the pounding hot water a long time, as if I could wash away memory and start over.

I reached the clinic before dawn, parked in the back, and dozed until someone came to open up. Out front, the protesters were already gathering, jubilant, taunting. They were obviously in contact with the group at my home and believed that I was successfully trapped there, unable to drive away because of the blocked driveway.

"No clinic today!" they jeered at the guards. "Your doctor won't make it today! No babies will die today!"

I called home to find that my fears had been justified. The driveway was completely blocked. The police still hadn't even begun to remove them from our property. The protesters had, however, rolled one barrel to the side enough to allow a police car to go pick up Sonja and then exit only after they had been convinced that I wasn't in the car as well. As soon as the car was out, the antis quickly put the barrel back in place. The remaining officer let them do whatever they wanted, waiting for reinforcements to come later in the morning.

Outside the clinic, 240 miles away from my home, the protesters continued celebrating their victory. I couldn't stand hearing them any more.

"That's enough," I muttered.

I opened the door at the front of the clinic and walked right out on the porch, stood there in my scrubs, and looked at the protesters, the suddenly silent protesters.

"I'm here!" I shouted. "I'm here, and there WILL be clinic today!" The look of shock and anger on their faces came really close to giving me some satisfaction.

Later that same day, between patients, I was called to the phone. It was the principal of Sonja's school. The tone of his voice when he called me by name told me immediately something was very wrong. "I just found Sonja in the hallway, surrounded by some of her friends, but crying." I could hear her in the background. Blood rushed to my head.

"What happened? What have they done to her?"

"She had a flyer crumpled in her hand," he said. "It has a picture of you. It calls you a murderer. It says that 'Sonja's mom kills unborn children.' I'm very sorry. We also found some of the troublemakers in the library looking at school yearbooks. I think they were looking for Sonja's picture, but we've gotten them out of the building."

"I'm so sorry, Sonja," I said, when I had her on the phone. "I'm so sorry."

"Mom," she said, her voice surprisingly firm. "Mom. Stop apologizing. It's okay. Really. I'm with friends. I'm alright. Stop worrying."

After I hung up, I sat numbly, Sonja's voice still in my head. I knew the antis were right about one thing: the support or lack of support by a physician's family is often the salient factor hanging in the balance, the single thing that weighs most heavily on the decision whether to continue providing abortion services. Getting to the doctor through his or her children or spouse is a despicable tactic, but an effective one.

I was sitting at the desk with the clinic director. While I was talking to Sonja, Jane was on another line. I could hear her saying, "No, Dr. Wicklund does not do media interviews."

"Who's that?" I interrupted.

"It's 60 *Minutes*," she said, covering the phone. "They want to do an interview. I told them you don't want to talk to them."

"Jane," I said, "tell them to hold on."

The protesters had invaded every corner of my life. They had violated me and the people I loved. They were making my work hell. They'd laid siege to my home, even entered my home. They were stalking me, confronting my daughter at her school, threatening us. Every shred of normalcy had been stripped from our lives. How could I, a media and mass communications virgin, hope to get the message to mainstream America that the protesters' claim of peaceful, prayerful protest was a blatant lie?

"Jane," I continued, "it's time. People have to know what's going on here. I'm ready to talk to *60 Minutes*. Give me the phone."

It was an impulsive decision but one I'd been subconsciously mulling over for some time. I had been doing my work, staying quiet, not broadcasting my commitment. Why should I have to, any more than an electrician or editor or brain surgeon has to make his or her work public? But as long as I kept it behind a curtain, hidden from view, the protesters could remain hidden and immune to consequences.

More important, bit by bit I was learning to trust people. When I spoke honestly, even to strangers, and even to people who weren't on the same philosophical page, what came back was support, understanding, even outrage. Was I ready to count on that response from a national audience of millions of people?

I would know soon enough.

In a matter of days one of the assistant producers had arrived with a sound and camera crew. The bulk of the filming took place in our home, at the clinic in Fargo, in airports, and on the road.

My interview with Lesley Stahl was arranged in a hotel room in Fargo. She'd been at the clinic much of the day, watching the protesters and police outside, absorbing the situation. She had been able to talk privately with several patients and had interviewed protesters.

In the hotel room it was difficult to relax and concentrate with the distraction of cameras and lights. The crew had a good chuckle over my lack of makeup. They asked me to powder my nose, and I had to borrow makeup from Lesley. That broke the ice, and I began to feel at ease.

Lesley established my background. We talked about my barricaded home, my work in regional clinics, the growing threat from protesters. We talked a little about my decision to take up this work and the price I paid for that commitment.

At one point Lesley asked, "Do you think there is a point at which it becomes so impossible you'll be forced to quit?"

"No," I said, immediately. "No, no," I repeated.

I hesitated for a moment. I thought of Sonja, of Randy, of Flower Grandma. They would all listen to this program.

"There are limits for everyone," I said. "I have to believe in my heart that even the protesters have their limits. Everyone has limits.

"At the same time," I added, "I'm cautious with my safety. I've handled firearms all my life. I carry a gun, and I know how to protect myself." That was for the protesters. Some of them would be watching, too.

Sonja held up remarkably well through all the turmoil and fear. When the *60 Minutes* piece aired four months later, she took it in stride. I was still reeling with emotions. I curled up in a blanket on the couch to watch, but my thoughts that night were of my Flower Grandma, home alone in her trailer with the flickering television. Alone with her memories.

The decision to go public to a huge audience was one of the most daunting choices I've ever faced, but in the end, it brought added protection for me and other physicians, as well as a heightened awareness to thousands of Americans about the real situation at clinics and the tactics of the protesters.

The segment drew tremendous support. I received more than a thousand letters. Less than a dozen were hateful or threatening. People poured out their hearts, shared their stories—stories of lives saved because of legal abortions and tragic accounts of lives lost in the days of illegal abortions.

"Just a vote of confidence and support," one typical letter read. "I am sixty-three years old—old enough to remember what it was like before *Roe v. Wade*. I don't want that world for my granddaughters. Do take care, and God bless you."

Nearer to home, neighbors I'd never met came out to offer help and support. New security measures were put in place in Sonja's school. The administrative staff, teachers, and Sonja's beloved swim coach all reached out in kindness. The local shelter volunteered to chauffeur Sonja to school and offered her safe haven if needed.

A parent of one of Sonja's friends called me at home to talk. She was mortified at what we, and especially Sonja, were enduring. She made it clear as we began our conversation that her personal beliefs were not necessarily pro-choice, but that having our family targeted and harassed was unacceptable.

As we talked more, she said that everyone should have the right to privacy in their home and that no one should be threatened for engaging in a legal activity. Before the talk was over, during which she offered their home as a refuge, we spoke more about choices. She ultimately agreed that no one should be able to make that choice for any woman. Not the government. Not a parent or husband or minister.

I pointed out that she was, by definition, pro-choice. In its simplest form all it means is that the woman gets to decide.

Never again would I feel as alone or exposed as I had before I spoke out publicly.

Then, a year after the airing of *60 Minutes*, the unthinkable happened.

I was taking a long overdue road trip with my dad. Just the two of us. We were driving through the Midwest on a sunny, glorious day to see Vince Gill and Mary Chapin Carpenter in concert in Iowa. It was March 9, 1993.

At a small gas station I decided to check in with the clinic I'd just opened in Montana. Stacey's voice was strained. "Call Jane in Fargo," she said. "You need to call Jane right now."

I remember everything about that gas station. The location of the phone along the inside south wall, tucked between the magazine rack and the car products. I remember the dull orange paint and the smell of the new linoleum, orange and blue stripes.

Jane's voice was almost a monotone, her words slow. "Sue," she said, "they've shot and killed an abortion doctor in Florida. Dr. Gunn. He's dead. Murdered."

I felt my knees buckle, and I sank to the floor, holding the phone, cord stretched, my jaw angled up to the receiver.

My mouth was open, but no words came out. I was slumped in that awkward position, shaking, my tears starting to flow when Dad walked in. He turned and looked down at me, startled.

"Shooting us, Dad. Abortion doctor. Gunned down. Dead. Oh no. No. No. No."

Dear Dr. Wicklund,

I want to begin this letter by apologizing that it has taken me two years to contact you. I am the woman who sat in your office more than two and a half years ago, crying and crying. You advised me to keep my baby, explaining that it would be more than I could handle emotionally to not keep her. You could not have been more correct. I prayed the night before I came to you and asked God to stop me if I was wrong. I wanted my baby so much. I had been in a four-year relationship; it had not been happy or stable (her father left when I was 5 months pregnant). My decision to come for an abortion was made with my mind, not my heart. My daughter was born on April 3, 2001. Rose weighed 8 lbs., 15 ounces. I cried for about five minutes after she was born; I knew in my heart that she was a girl. I now have one girl and one boy. I purchased our first home last July and we love it! I want you to know that I will be forever grateful to you. It is very possible that I would not have survived the wrong decision.

Former Patient

— chapter seven

Just a month before the first murder of an abortion provider, I had opened up my own private clinic in Bozeman, Montana. So many events in my life have come about because of serendipitous events. The opportunity to operate my own clinic was no exception.

In late November of 1992 I was working at the clinic in Fargo. Fargo Women's Health Organization was housed in an old, two-story wood building. It had been a single family home at one time, then converted into a clinic. It was mid-morning, but we had been unable to start seeing patients because of a large protest. Women were having a hard time getting in or were reluctant to attempt breaching the wall of confusion made up of protesters, police, security personnel, volunteer escorts, and media.

Most of our staff was standing in the waiting room on the second floor, watching out windows. Different factions would dominate the scene at different times. Watching the ebb and flow of the action was like seeing a war unfold. I had seen enough and retreated down to the main floor to finish setting up the procedure rooms.

The phone was ringing, and no one was answering it. I was sure the receptionist was on the other line, but the ringing wouldn't stop, and although I hardly ever take calls, I finally answered it.

"Fargo Women's Health. How can I help you?"

"Could I please speak with your doctor? The woman doctor? The one I saw on *60 Minutes*?"

Because we get so many crank calls and even death threats, I was reluctant to identify myself. Still, there was something about this caller's voice that was not threatening.

"May I ask what you'd like to speak to her about?"

"Certainly," he replied. "I am also an abortion provider and have a clinic in Bozeman, Montana. I just wanted to give her my support and encourage her to keep working."

With that, Dr. Balice and I delved into a twenty-minute conversation about the challenges, joys, twisted logistics, and everyday reality of providing abortion services. We talked about being marginalized in the medical community, about our resolve not to give up in spite of the threats. We agreed on the importance of supporting each other and our other colleagues.

Toward the end of our conversation, he mentioned that he was past retirement age and anxious to spend some time on the ski slopes. He had been unable to find anyone willing to take over his practice, but he refused to close the doors. He knew that the protesters would take undeserved credit for ending abortion services in Bozeman.

I was speechless.

"Excuse me," I mumbled. "Did you say you wanted someone to come and work for you?"

"No," he replied. "I am looking for someone to completely take over. Someone to buy my clinic."

I immediately knew that this was my chance, a chance I had been fantasizing about for some time. I'd looked into it enough to know that the financial risk was tremendous, the responsibility and increased exposure sobering, and the consequences for my family substantial.

But I also understood that owning and running my own facility would allow me to elevate counseling and recovery to the level I had always believed necessary, to pick everything from the décor to the music we played, and to handle each aspect of the many financial and ethical decisions without interference.

I told him I would fly out within a week. Before clinic was finally in full swing later that morning, I had already made the necessary arrangements to travel to Bozeman. I still had three days of work to focus on before the trip, but that didn't keep me from daydreaming about providing more than just abortions. Pregnancy planning and prevention, prenatal care and births, annual exams, well-woman care—abortions are only one facet of the services available in a clinic that truly provides choices for women.

I had been doing abortions full time for less than five years but was already a veteran through working in five clinics in three states, packing in an intense amount of frontline experience. In that brief time, I had learned so much from counselors and educators and clinic directors who were all dedicated to their patients. More to the point, I had learned from the hundreds of women who presented themselves, and their life situations, to me over that time. Now I had an opportunity to take the best of each clinic, along with my accumulating experience, and fashion it into a facility with my name and style behind it.

I'm the first to admit that I like being in control. I don't think that is a bad trait in most situations, and in the case of providing abortion services, the doctor is the one ultimately responsible. It made complete sense for me to manage the entire experience, not just the procedure.

As the doctor actually performing the abortion, the one who physically removes an embryo or fetus from the pregnant woman's uterus, I had better be sure this is truly what she has chosen of her own free will. The clinic staff is a team. It has to be. The receptionist, the counselors, the lab techs, the surgical assistants, the nurses, and the doctor all have to be on the same page.

Still, I am the one who ends a potential human life. I am the one who lives in fear of performing an abortion on someone who will later regret it. I am the one asking a woman to lie back so that I can begin the procedure. I had better be listening to her unspoken fears and paying attention to her body language. I have to be tuned to the questions that signal ambivalence.

I have to know the subtle shades of difference between "I want," "I need," and "I should" for each patient on every day, no matter what else is going on to complicate or confuse the issue.

It was one of those confusing issues, and my lack of attention, that resulted in an abortion I will always regret having done.

The patient and her husband came together to the clinic. It was during one of the first years I was working full-time, and that clinic did not have an ultrasound. We estimated the stage of a patient's pregnancy based on her last normal menstrual period (LMP) and by pelvic exam to determine the size of the uterus.

When the patient and I reviewed her medical history prior to the abortion, I asked my usual question, "Are you absolutely sure of your decision to have this abortion?" She was obviously sad, but very clear in her decision and had the complete support of her husband.

"Yes, I want to do this," she said. "There is no way I could possibly carry this pregnancy full term. I just cannot have this baby."

With hindsight, I should have asked a few more questions. "Why can't you have this baby?" for example. I knew there were no medical reasons, but what was driving her? There were no clues in the notes from the counselor, and I didn't probe further.

The patient was a large woman. Due to her size, the pelvic exam was difficult and less accurate than I liked. Her history suggested she was about eight weeks since her last menstrual period. I could tell that we were within two weeks of that. She was certainly no more than ten weeks, and probably less. I continued with an uneventful abortion. The procedure took about five minutes, and she handled it well.

We moved her to the recovery room, and the tissue we removed from the uterus was taken to the lab for evaluation. We always examine the products of conception

(POC), both to confirm the stage of pregnancy and to look for any abnormal tissue. On examination of the POC, it was obvious that she was actually around ten weeks LMP, meaning she had conceived at least two weeks earlier than expected by her history. I always tell the patients if we find something unexpected.

Upon entering the recovery room, I sat down next to the patient and asked how she was coping.

"Fine. Total relief, really. If I had given birth to that baby, it would have been a constant reminder of the rape. I have always been very against abortion, but in this case it was the only thing I could do."

I was holding my breath. This was new information to me. Was the embryo we just aborted the rapist's or her husband's? I stifled a gasp. Questions raced through my head. When was the rape? I had to tell her what I had found, but what if . . . ?

"Mrs. P., I don't know when the rape was, but after looking at the tissue that came out of your uterus, I need to tell you that you conceived at least two weeks earlier than we had estimated."

The color drained out of her face. The lines around her eyes and mouth began to change and contract. She kept moving her eyes from me to the door, as if she was about to bolt.

"What? What do you mean? When did I get pregnant? I got pregnant from the rape, right? Right?"

I tried to stand, to go to the desk to get the wheel that we use to determine weeks of pregnancy and most likely conception dates, but my legs wouldn't work. I broke into a sweat. The nurse sitting at the desk had figured out the situation and handed me the wheel. She and I looked at each other, trying to hide the look of horror in our faces.

Together we went over the facts, the date of the rape, the stage of the pregnancy as evidenced by the POC. The pregnancy was clearly not a result of the rape.

"Oh my God, what have we done?" she choked.

Mrs. P was inconsolable. I had another staff member get her husband from the waiting room, and I had to tell him what we had learned. In a gesture that would have horrified a malpractice lawyer, I apologized over and over. The three of us cried together. This pregnancy, this baby, would have been very welcomed and loved had they known it was theirs. But now it was ended, and I felt responsible. I was responsible.

We spent lots of time, the three of us, trying to comfort each other. Before they left, we exchanged home phone numbers, promised to talk again soon. They never blamed me or threatened legal action against me or the clinic. We all had counseling to deal with the guilt and sadness over the event. More than anything, I learned to never assume anything, to always ask the questions in my heart, to listen to what wasn't said, to pay attention to my intuition, and to never do an abortion without having an ultrasound first.

Another thing I learned from that patient and her partner: how great is the gift of forgiveness. I was still trying to forgive the doctor who did my abortion years ago. Not because I had any regrets, but because of the terrible way I was treated. Every single day I worked, and with each patient I treated, I remembered that abortion. At the core, I was determined to make my patients' experiences better than mine had been.

A clinic facility that expressed my priorities, my values, and my style was taking shape in my imagination when I flew into Bozeman. The plane banked over the Bridger Mountains. The broad Gallatin River valley spread below, surrounded by mountain ranges. I could barely contain my excitement.

Two summers before I had visited Montana for the first time, joining a group of friends for a horse pack trip in the Bob Marshall Wilderness. I had spent eight days in the backcountry. Eight days free of protesters. Eight days away from television, away from news of the outside world. There, I gained a sense of peace I had never known before. I recognized that the mountains offered me a refuge, a place where I could renew myself, and I had dreamed of that possibility ever since. In Bozeman I could do the work I loved and have the solace I needed out my back door.

The airport had just two gates. All the faces were friendly and open. Walking from the plane into the main building I could feel the cold, dry air—a welcome change from the thick humidity in the Midwest. I felt as if I were home, as if the mountains were holding their ridges out to me in an embrace.

Dr. Balice met me at the baggage claim. A small man with a big grin and a cowboy hat, he was gracious and talkative and excited. We drove right to the clinic, and I immediately saw some of its advantages. It was in a building with many other offices: a dentist, an accountant, a few doctors, the American Red Cross, a surgery center, a pharmacy, and a medical lab. Being in a building with other businesses would prevent the clinic from becoming an isolated target. Protesters would have a harder time singling out women entering the building for abortion services. The activity and variety would make it difficult for them to harass and pinpoint the staff and patients. From the first, I liked it.

When I walked through the door, I noticed a stained glass panel made by Dr. Balice. But then I looked past everything else and started to sketch in my own clinic. I could imagine the comfortable chairs and alternative magazines in the waiting room. I could see Carol Griggs's prints on the walls and hear Tracy Chapman music. I would have coffee and juice and snacks available. Everything would be arranged to help calm and reassure patients, encouraging them to be informed partners in the process.

The clinic was small. As I walked through, I brainstormed the layout I'd design. A room with nice windows had great potential for a counseling space. I would furnish it with a small couch, a rocker, and a small desk. Maybe I'd install a fish tank for a focal point when discussions were tough. The view out the third floor window framed the peaks of the Bridger Range, and that high up, curtains wouldn't be needed.

Two other rooms would be the exam and procedure rooms, with a small lab adjacent. I could see remodeling possibilities that would provide a separate entrance/exit into the recovery room for patient privacy. I would get overstuffed couches that pushed back into recliners so patients could get comfortable while recovering. It would be a quiet room with more to eat, lots to read, and an ambiance designed to provide support and healing.

Within twenty-four hours of my arrival, Dr. Balice and I had come to an agreement on terms and timing. I would come back shortly after Christmas. I planned to open my doors in February of 1993. I was beside myself with excitement, leavened with more than a little apprehension.

Neither Randy nor Sonja had any intention of being uprooted, and until we knew the clinic would actually be a success, it didn't make sense for them to move anyway. Randy had just finished college and begun an engineering career. Sonja had more than two years of high school left. She was completely engaged in her education and friends. My work had asked so much of her already. The last thing I could expect was for her to leave home.

I needed a place to live in Bozeman three nights a week. The other days I would come back to the Midwest and continue to work at two clinics I had been serving for four years. I'd get one day a week with my family, if everything went without a hitch.

The month of January was crammed with preparing for my own medical practice—legal considerations, writing protocols, gathering medical supplies and equipment, and finding a place to live. For a time I felt, and in fact was, incredibly isolated. I had few friends or contacts and lived a kind of obsessive existence in which my clinic became my central and only focus.

In mid-January I found a small apartment just six blocks away from the medical building. I took every precaution I could think of to keep the location a secret. I never walked directly to the apartment. I'd walk a circuitous route, usually heading out in the opposite direction, making stops along the way, coming and going at different times. Sometimes I'd duck into a restaurant, sit alone at a table for an hour, then leave by the back door. I never spoke to any of the other tenants in the apartment complex, which is completely contrary to my nature. I longed to make small talk, meet people who smiled as we passed outside the building, find out about the town, live normally.

Often as not, the easiest thing was to spend the night at the office. I was afraid to walk home alone after dark. I had so much to do. I slept on the recliner in the recovery room. Staff would bring me coffee and bagels in the morning.

Most of Dr. Balice's staff stayed on to help me get things up and running, but did not intend to stay long term. That meant hiring new people. The responsibility of handpicking my staff was as exciting as it was daunting. The first position I filled was the clinic manager. The woman I hired was perfect. Stacy was dedicated, professional, determined, and excellent with patients. She also had a great instinct when hiring other new staff, and soon we had a team assembled I felt comfortable and confident with.

Mountain Country Women's Clinic opened its doors on February 2, 1993. From the start, counseling formed the core emphasis of patient care. I had always been at my best with one-to-one interactions, and I had hired staff who were intuitive and committed to the same style. We worked as a unit, sharing responsibilities from front desk to lab to clean up, with counseling being a focus for all of us.

No patient was turned away for financial reasons, but each staff member had complete veto power regarding the provision of services for any individual patient. Often we spent hours on a single patient before ever getting to the procedure. Sometimes we never would get to the procedure.

In counseling sessions, immersed in women's stories and dilemmas, we heard over and over again about the real difficulties and choices they faced. With each case, each situation, we also learned about ourselves. Most important, we began to understand that above all, we simply had to listen.

As always, the patients kept me strong. Within weeks of opening our doors, there was already a handful of women whose experiences and circumstances reaffirmed my philosophy. I had a business to run, and the financial burden kept me awake some nights, but I knew I was doing everything I possibly could to keep our patients both physically and emotionally safe. It became the most important and rewarding part of my work. I knew, from my own experiences, how essential it was to be fully informed, and I could see daily, in the looks of gratitude and relief, what it meant to the women we served. That was the bottom line that mattered.

It wasn't uncommon for a woman to return three or four times before she'd feel comfortable with her decision. In the first month of my new practice I handled one such patient: forty years old, a successful career woman, torn between her ticking biological clock and the present circumstances of her life.

"Deep down I think I'll regret having this abortion," she said at one point during her first visit. "I know I'm getting to an age where I have to decide about having children. But then when I think about everything else—my relationship, my work—I can't imagine having a child."

As soon as she said that, I knew we wouldn't be doing an abortion, not that day anyway. But we talked nearly an hour longer. Everything about her body language communicated her indecision, her ambiguity.

"Do you think it's the situation, your circumstances, that you'll regret, or is it the abortion itself?"

No response. A shrug of shoulders.

"That's a big distinction. You need to sort that out. This is not the time for a snap decision. Work it through more. Give it the time you need."

"I feel so terribly irresponsible!" she said.

"Look," I said, taking her by the shoulders, "it's the people who don't think things through, who make no plans and ignore reality until they're really stuck and then can't cope—they are the irresponsible ones.

"You've met us now. You've seen the clinic and how we work. Take your money and go sort this out. Come back if you need to."

Two days later she returned.

"I just want to do it," she said. "All this thinking is driving me crazy. Let's just do it and be done with it."

"No. This is irreversible. We never 'just do it.'" I sent her on her way again.

But when she returned a third time, a week later, I could see the difference in her even before she said a word. Gone was the cocoon she had wrapped herself in earlier. Gone were the nervous, fidgety mannerisms, the hesitation before tough questions.

"I'm absolutely sure now," she told me. "I regret my situation, but this is the right choice." Her eyes held mine.

"Is this your head talking now, or your heart?" I asked, although I already knew the answer.

"My heart," she said, with absolute certainty in her voice and in her manner.

I had devoted three counseling sessions to this single patient. Three unpaid sessions, from a business point of view. But there is more than one consequence in these cases. The financial one pales in comparison to the human, emotional one.

That patient expressed her gratitude when she left the clinic. "Thank you for making me wait and work through all the things I was struggling with on this choice," she said. "I'd have been a wreck if you had done the abortion the first time I came in."

Many times the counseling involves more than just the patient. Parents, boyfriends, or husbands are frequently very involved in the dialogue, but the decision is still ultimately the woman's.

Another day I spent nearly an hour on the phone with the mother of a young pregnant girl. She had been calling all the clinics in the region to get a sense for which would be the best for her daughter.

They lived in a small Wyoming city. Their daughter, the way the mother described her, reminded me of Sonja. She was a responsible kid, at the top of her school class, active in sports and other activities, busy with her friends.

"She went to a movie one night," the mother told me. "We always insisted that she walk home with friends in the neighborhood when she was out late, and she always did. But this one night her girlfriends were in a hurry, and my daughter told them not to bother. It was only a few blocks. She knew that if she called we would come and get her . . . "

After a silence, the mother continued. "She was raped in those few blocks. On the way home my daughter was raped.

"But worse than that, she felt so terrible and so guilty, as if it were her fault! She couldn't bring herself to tell us this awful thing. She couldn't tell us.

"Last week I noticed that the supplies for her period hadn't been touched for a while. I really wasn't sure how long. When I asked her if something was wrong with her period, she broke down in tears. It was only then that she told me, and by that time she knew she was probably pregnant."

I could hear the emotion in her voice, threatening to break through. "How overdue is your daughter?" I asked, moving us on.

We discussed in detail the process our clinic went through with each patient. By the time we finished she had decided to make an appointment. I insisted, however, that the daughter make her own appointment, stressing that we do abortions at the request of the woman, not a parent or husband. The mother understood what I was saying and put the daughter on the phone.

We had a brief discussion, long enough for me to confirm the things the mother had told me, and for me to be convinced that she indeed wanted to end this pregnancy. She had, in fact, been making calls herself, inquiring about how to get an abortion.

"Is it all right if my parents both come?"

"Of course it is. That is the way it should be," I replied.

They arrived within days, after a six-hour drive. All three of them were well dressed, neatly groomed, polite, exuding an air of prosperity and a careful control over their emotions.

While the daughter began her counseling with one of my staff, and with her permission, I asked her parents to join me in my office.

"I know you are concerned," I began. "And I want to fully explain the procedure your daughter will go through, if that's her decision." The man looked a little startled at the possibility his daughter might not elect the abortion. "It sounds, in this case, as if Ellen is pretty clear. But it's very important that we reach a complete understanding with each patient, and that the choice is an informed one." He nodded.

I went through the technicalities of the procedure, at one point drawing a diagram of the uterus on a notepad to illustrate the stage of her pregnancy. I could feel the father's growing agitation as I continued. I wondered how much a part of all this he had been, whether he had fully dealt with his own feelings.

The mother had a few questions after I finished, and then we sat together in silence.

"I come from a family that never showed emotion," the father broke the quiet. "If you had a problem, you dealt with it. You didn't go burdening others with your trivial difficulties."

His wife had turned to him, but he was staring off through the window.

"Now I see that my family is the same way." His hand came to his face, ran quickly through his hair. "I feel so ashamed that my little girl couldn't tell us that this, this criminal, hateful, violent thing had happened to her.

"She tried to take care of it all alone, thinking it would be a burden to us, that somehow this crime was her fault and that it would be better," he pounded his hand softly on his thigh, "that it would be better if we didn't know."

His voice broke. His wife put her hand on his. I moved closer. "I love her so much," he was openly crying now. All of us were. "I love her so much, and I am so terribly ashamed that she wouldn't come to us for help, that she kept this to herself."

He turned to his wife, and they embraced. She comforted him, cried with him. I wondered if he had ever sobbed in her arms before, if he had cried in his adult life.

"If we hadn't discovered her pregnancy, she might have buried it from us always," he said through tears.

When he had collected himself a bit, I left to check on their daughter.

"How are you doing?" I asked her.

"Better," she admitted. "I finally understand that the only thing I did wrong that night was to walk home alone. It isn't my fault I was raped. It isn't my fault I am pregnant."

"No, it certainly isn't," I said. "But you aren't alone. Many women feel the way you did. That they are somehow responsible for being the victim of a sex crime."

"I just wish my father could understand," she said.

"I think he does," I reassured her.

She shook her head.

"He's in the other room right now, crying in your mother's arms." She looked at me in disbelief. "He told me how much he loves you, how terrible he feels about all this."

"No," she said. "I know he loves me, but he'd never say it. He's never said that!"

"I think maybe he should come in here. I think you two need to talk."

I left the room and returned with her parents, leading her father in first. She saw his tear-streaked face, hesitated just a moment, and then went to him. They held each other as if they hadn't hugged since she was an infant. This man who never showed emotion, who had never told his sixteen-year-old child that he loved her—he held her now as if he would never stop, crying anew, kissing her hair, saying again and again how much he loved her, how sorry he was, and what a gift she was in his life.

All three of them came back out together, laughing their relief, looking at each other with different eyes and obviously aware of some hurdle they had just cleared as a family.

After that session, the abortion procedure was truly anti-climactic. The mother stayed with her daughter throughout, held her hand much of the time. All of them sat together in the recovery room, listening attentively to our after-care instructions.

By the time they left, they were changed people; the barriers had evaporated. I believed that no terrible secret would ever divide them again.

I walked them to the stairs to say good-bye. The young woman and her mother started down, but the father turned to me again, started to hold out his hand, then pulled me into an embrace.

"Thank you," he whispered, his voice fierce with emotion. "Thank you for keeping my daughter safe."

My experience with that family reaffirmed my belief in the importance of talking things through, allowing a story to unfold and paying attention to intuitive cues that so often lead to breakthroughs. The powerful experience these people shared had nothing to do with parental notification laws or twenty-four-hour waiting periods. It was the result of their commitment to each other, the opportunity to fully express their feelings, and the force of events to catalyze a revelation.

Some days women come to the clinic saying they want an abortion, but nothing they say or do convinces us that the decision is whole-hearted or genuine. Everything about them screams no, regardless of what their voices say.

Some of them are being threatened by partners or parents. Some just can't see any other way out of a bad situation. In either case, we have to be cautious. I would rather have someone be very angry at me, even to the point of taking legal action against me, for *not* doing an abortion, than for doing an abortion she later regrets. It isn't uncommon to get a letter or picture in the mail, as much as a year later, thanking us for our refusal.

Most women, by the time they arrive at a clinic, are very clear in their decision. They have been tormented by the dilemmas they face for days or weeks, sometimes months. They need the counseling sessions to simply clarify and solidify their convictions.

Even then, it can be a murky process. It is one thing for a woman to decide on a course of action, but sometimes quite another to truly own that decision. Some patients are very adept at pulling me in, as if they want me to recommend an abortion so they can feel more removed from that responsibility.

"I've been smoking and drinking alcohol while I've been pregnant," they might confide in me. "Don't you think it's best to have an abortion rather than risk a birth defect?"

"Sure, it's a risk," I'll throw back at them, "but there's no way to predict the outcome. What if you hadn't been smoking or drinking? Would you want to go through with your pregnancy?"

Almost always, when they are honest, they'll admit that it wouldn't make a difference. They simply want me to validate their decision, and perhaps assume some of their burden.

Once in a while the simple question I ask each patient just before starting the procedure will bring out startling information I hadn't anticipated.

I had a patient once who seemed as calm and ordinary as they come. She could have been Sonja's grade school teacher or the woman behind the counter at the grocery store. We went through her history, and she received counseling, had her lab tests, and completed all the paperwork. None of us picked up on any tension or unspoken agenda. She was sitting on the exam table, and we were about to start, when I asked the questions I always ask.

"Are you absolutely sure you want this abortion? Is there anyone pushing you or telling you to be here? Is this really your decision?"

"If I couldn't have this abortion, I'd kill myself," she said, voice flat and matter-of-fact.

"What?" I asked, stunned, but completely believing her.

"The man I've been living with for the last two years is abusive. I have two children. We're trying to get him out of our lives, but he refuses to leave and even threatened me with a gun two days ago. I filed for a restraining order yesterday."

She paused, gathered herself, then went on.

"My girl and I are very close. She's fourteen now. We talk a lot, and she understands so much for her age. Too much. When I found out I was pregnant, I wanted to tell her, to see what she thought about it.

"We were sitting together on the couch. She was half facing me, but as soon as she understood what I was telling her, she pushed herself off like she couldn't get away fast enough. She started backing away from me. Backing across the room, her face all twisted up and her frantic voice shouting at me.

'Mother,' she said. 'Mother, you can't have his baby! NO! NO! We'll never get rid of him then! It would look like him! It would talk like him! Walk like him! Be like him! Mother, it would act like he does. It would hurt me the way he hurts me! NO! NO!'"

By the time the woman finished she was shaking. Tears streaked her face. "Do you understand me? Do you see why I could never have this man's baby?"

As I did her abortion, all I could think about was this woman's life, her two children, and that abusive man. It was hard to focus on the technical work of the procedure. Thoughts kept sweeping into my head. What would she have done if safe, legal abortion hadn't been an option? What would her life and her daughter's life have been like?

Something else was working on me. She had gone through all the required and routine steps at the clinic. Only when I asked her these last questions had all of this come out. Why? And was it important that she verbalize all this for me anyway? Did I need to be privy to this information?

Both the patient and I were rather quiet through the short time it took to end the pregnancy. Each of us was deep in our own, private thoughts. When she was dressed and headed for recovery, I stopped her and asked her to stay a minute longer. I apologized to her, thinking I had perhaps pushed her too far, gotten too personal with my inquiry.

"No, oh no." She shook her head. "I am so glad I got that out of my system. When I was telling you about my daughter's reaction to all of this, I realized how much I felt the same. Saying it all out loud completely took away all doubt I might have had. No, I am so glad you asked the question you did. Thank you."

When I leave the clinic after a day of work, there are patients who stay in my thoughts. Often it is the ambivalent woman we send away. I hope we have given her the tools she needs to come to a clear decision. I hope that she understands we all have choices. We at the clinic have a right, even an obligation, to refuse an abortion if we don't believe a patient really wants it.

My thoughts might be with a fourteen-year-old who couldn't even comprehend how she got pregnant but, thanks to our educators, now understands the mystery. I think about how we affect family dynamics, like the sixteen-year-old rape victim. It is a tremendous satisfaction to know that she and her father will communicate in a healthier way, and that we helped make that difference by opening the doors to honest dialogue.

All of this, of course—the way I think about patients and their outcomes, the way I approach a patient when I first meet her, my voice, my questions, my empathy—comes from my own experiences. It is shaped by the way my abortion unfolded in 1976, by the difficult decisions I have had to make, and by what I have learned from patients and staff and life. I hold these things in me every day. They come with me into every counseling session. They are who I am.

Missoula
Feb. 17, 1993

Dear Susan Wicklund,

As promised in my Feb. 16 letter,
you're now hearing from me again.

We will shut you down, you murdering butcher.
How dare you kill unborn Americans! What gives
you the right! How would you like to be torn limb
from limb in your mother's womb, your head
crushed, and then thrown on a garbage dump?

Or, how would you like to be slowly tortured to
death by suffocating and burning by saline?

You murderess. We will end your vile practice,
you cold-blooded murderess!!

How many babies have you murdered in your
"illustrious" career? 100? 500? 1,000?
Proud of it, are you, you reptile?

Stop the killing. Stop murdering
innocent children. Until next time.

Mike Ross

— chapter eight

The woman behind the counter looked at me as if I were her definition of a really bad day. She was confused and exasperated. This was a simple transaction she could accomplish with her eyes closed.

"Look," I repeated. "I need to have the utility bills sent to the Mountain Country Women's Clinic, not the apartment, and I can't have my name on it."

"Okay," she said, sighing. "You are the person living at this address, correct?"

"Yes, we've established that. But I can't have the bill sent there. I can't have my name associated with that address. I can't even have my name on the account."

"That's not possible," she said, her voice flat and final.

"It has to be possible," I said, just as adamant.

We stared at each other.

My turn to sigh. "This is my situation," I said, leaning toward her across the counter. "I'm the doctor who owns that clinic. We offer women's reproductive health care. We also perform abortions. There are people stalking me, threatening me. I don't like it one bit, but I have to be thinking about that all the time. I can't just set up an account like most people. They will track me down, find where I live. Then, who knows?"

"Oh," she said.

Her expression softened. She went very silent. "Give me a minute," she said. "Let me think about how to do this."

The move to Bozeman was exciting, even exhilarating, but it was fraught with complications and danger. I had to take precautions worthy of a witness protection placement in order to stay off the radar of anti-abortion zealots.

At that time, there were no anti-stalking laws in Montana. I could be followed and approached with impunity. By the time any law enforcement could legally become engaged, it would be too late. I kept my Minnesota driver's license to avoid having my local address on record. I had an unlisted phone number. My checking account was tied to the clinic address.

Everything was complicated by that reality. By now I was used to feeling like prey, used to watching my back, but in Bozeman I was truly alone. No family. No friends. Totally exposed.

Mine was a life of constant airport runs, different beds, different colleagues, different offices, different vehicles and streets. I was always on guard, listening for the wrong voice, watching for the eyes that meant trouble, checking the rearview mirror, never knowing who would be on the other end of a telephone call.

Sometimes it felt completely unreal, silly, overblown. The shenanigans I had to go through were ridiculous. But I had no choice.

I wouldn't allow the janitorial service to clean the offices. My staff and I handled that chore. When I spent the night, I never turned any lights on in rooms facing the street, never even went in those rooms. I bought a tiny television and kept it in the box, hidden under a table. Some nights I'd pull it out, make popcorn in the microwave, and let the mindless TV shows keep me company.

Always, Michael Ross hovered in the background, a forbidding predator. The day the clinic opened I started receiving his threatening letters. They came two or three at a time. He would scrawl out descriptions of how he was going to kill me—tear off my arms and legs, squish my head and watch the brains come out like Jell-O, set me on fire and listen to me scream. Day after day they sat in the pile of mail, his distinctive, handwritten scrawl a beacon of hatred.

He actually signed the letters, but the law enforcement people I contacted wouldn't investigate. Written threats were not a punishable offense, they told me. My office manager collected them, opened and read them, filed them. She developed a sense for when to keep the letters from me, days when she picked up my frazzled, stressed-out vibes. In the first month, sixty-three of his letters came in the mail.

The clinic could not be targeted directly by protesters, but they would be on the street and sidewalk in front of the building, carrying their signs, watching for me, trying to identify likely patients. People who arrived for dentist appointments, visits to their accountant, or to give blood at the American Red Cross and even customers at the pharmacy would have to deal with the ugly signs and rhetoric.

By and large, most of the other tenants in the building were at least not hostile. An investment broker and another physician in the building went out of their way to visit and offer assistance. Of course, another tenant posted a Right to Life poster on their office window. Although I didn't venture out to socialize, I was very grateful to those who offered friendship.

By the same token, people unknown to me came and went all the time. They could be in my hallway, in the restroom on our floor, coming and going in the elevator right by the door to the clinic. I never knew who might be there to harass my patients or target me.

Within several weeks of opening I was invited to a private slide show. Some local people were sharing their canoe adventure in northern Canada. The man who invited me had given me a book by another Bozeman couple who had spent more than a year in the wilds of Canada, paddling across the continent and spending the winter in a remote log cabin. I was completely engrossed by the idea of these extended wilderness expeditions. Right then, nothing sounded better than to escape to some place wild and pure, some place far removed from protesters, death threats, airport corridors, clinics, and the media.

Yes, I was in Montana, surrounded by clear air and mountain views. The fact was, however, that I was so occupied with the clinic, my work, and my vulnerability that my world stayed small. For all the opportunity I had to embrace Montana, I might as well have been in New York City.

That winter evening, with a snowstorm blowing outside, surrounded by friendly people, I sat alone, watching the images of water and boats and campsites in the middle of vast country. It was all I could do not to break into tears. I thought of the book I had been reading, the experiences these people shared. I was deeply envious of their ability to craft a life full of adventure.

During a break in the slides, I was introduced to a couple. It didn't take me long to realize that they were the people in the book. I connected with them immediately. Marypat was eight months pregnant with their second child. Their first son had been conceived on one of their extended northern canoe expeditions. We talked about her experience using a midwife for her first delivery and her plans to continue that practice.

I was thrilled to be around someone with a planned and desired pregnancy. Marypat had such positive energy. She and Al, her husband, were completely dedicated to incorporating adventure into their family life. Before the evening was over, we made plans to have supper together soon.

The next six weeks were outrageous. Schedule chaos was a familiar syndrome, but this was a new level. Within two months of opening the clinic I'd fallen into a routine where every week, on Wednesday, I flew back to the Midwest after work to share a short night home with Randy and Sonja. Too short to reconnect much beyond hearing about Sonja's school life and Randy's work before dropping into bed. Early on Thursday morning, I'd fly to another clinic to finish out the week.

Most Saturdays I worked at a different clinic. Finally, on Sunday, I could sleep in, share a late family breakfast, then start in on laundry, bills, chores, trying to catch up. Sonja, as a high school sophomore, took my place in the household, sharing the cleaning, cooking, chores, and laundry with Randy. She took it in stride, but I felt deep guilt for the burden my work placed on her and for my absence in her daily life.

On Sunday mornings I made a point of cooking breakfast and almost always burned the bacon. When Sonja noticed me bustling around in the kitchen, she quickly learned to make a beeline for the closet, where she'd unhook the alarm system. The smoke alarm was combined with the burglar alarm, a security system we'd had installed in the old farmhouse. Another reminder of the underlying threat we all tried to ignore.

Too soon it was time to drive to the airport for the late flight to Bozeman. I couldn't let myself think about how frenzied it all was and how tough it was on my marriage and my relationship with Sonja. If I fell into that trap, I'd never climb out again. Each week before leaving again I held Sonja tight in my arms, smelled her hair. Randy and I would hug, look at each other, and make every effort to ignore the distance my work was putting between us.

Back in the Bozeman airport, a security person met me. The protesters were often in attendance too. Gone was the initial impression of this small, friendly western airport. It had become another place to fear and dread as I came up the ramp from the plane. I'd made arrangements with airport officials to exit the plane directly onto the tarmac when the protesters were particularly riled up. My security person picked me up in a protected lot. On our drive back to the apartment we'd make a few evasive turns and loops, watch for cars behind us.

The next morning it started again. On Monday I'd take my roundabout walk to the clinic and open up. It was lonely, hectic, numbing, but the clinic was thriving, and that kept me going. Once inside the office, I loved my work and the freedom to create an atmosphere that reflected my personality and priorities. Without that satisfaction, I could never have pulled it off.

Airplanes became my auxiliary office. Flying across the country, I wrote in my journal, thought about problems, read books. Sometimes I fell into deep, strange sleeps full of dream collages from my scattered life.

Water and Sky, the book by the couple I'd met, took me away to that wilderness place full of wind and river current and isolation. I savored every page. I read the last chapter on a flight from Bozeman to Minneapolis. In the story, Marypat and Al had arrived at a tiny town at the end of their fourteen-month journey. A plane would soon fly them back to civilization. Marypat wandered away to a nearby rise. She mourned the end of their yearlong immersion in nature, questioned their return.

Sitting on the plane, I was completely transported. I became Marypat. I was caught up in the power and vastness of this experience, resisting the end, fundamentally torn between realities. I ached to be in that wilderness place. The flight attendant shook my shoulder, asked if I was okay. Only then did I realize that I was sobbing.

I'd lived in Bozeman long enough by then to make some contacts. I had been to Al and Marypat's house for supper. There were a few people who made a point of getting me out once in awhile. A lawyer I'd met invited me out for some late night in-line skating on Main Street when the weather permitted. It was completely against city ordinance but also an incredible release to be out late at night cruising down sidewalks, doing laps around parking lots. More than once we had to skate in the front door of a bar, through the crowd of people, and out the back door to escape apprehension. It was giddy and exhilarating, but also another reminder that my life was on the edge.

One week in early March my schedule changed. It was the weekend Dad and I traveled to the concert in Iowa, when Dr. Gunn was murdered in Florida by anti-abortionist Michael Griffin. I stayed an extra night in Minnesota before flying back to Montana on Monday.

Tom, my security guard, picked me up and drove me to the apartment. It was a ground floor unit, the door directly off the driveway. Right away I saw that the outside light was off. I always left it on. It could have burned out, but I was immediately on alert. Tom and I walked up to the door together. I got out my key, but it was already open. Even the deadbolt was unlocked.

We looked at each other. Tom took the lead, shouldered into the hallway. I stuck close behind. Nothing was disturbed in the tiny kitchen/sitting area, but a trail of muddy boot prints led out from the bedroom. We followed them to the window by the bed. It had been pried open. Whoever broke in made no attempt at secrecy. On the bedside stand they had left a stack of anti-abortion pamphlets.

I tried to process the possibilities and smother my fear. They had located me. Presumably, they also knew my routine. Had someone been here in the past twenty-four hours, when I would normally be home? Had they come in the window the night before, expecting to find me?

I kept a loaded pistol in bed with me. If I had woken to an intruder, that gun would have been in their face. I could have killed someone. The possibility was a tremendous burden, even if it would have been a justifiable instance of self-defense. At the same time, this was a fundamental, bone-chilling violation of my space, my privacy, my safety. It made me angry, frightened, resentful.

Clearly, whenever the break-in occurred, it was intended to put me on notice. I turned and fled, taking nothing, pushing past Tom, almost running for the car.

Tom locked up the apartment and drove me to a phone. I called Al and Marypat. They had mentioned a guest room in their basement that I could use whenever I felt the need. My apartment had become a crime scene. I would report it to the police in the morning.

That week, one of Michael Ross's letters referred to Dr. Gunn's killing. "I wonder if a similar fate might come to you," he wrote.

Even armed with that evidence, I couldn't get the attention of the local law enforcement people. The best they could offer was to suggest that I apply for a concealed weapons permit. In order to get it, I had to demonstrate that

I was competent with a firearm and with a pistol in particular. I went with one of the officers to the shooting range and outscored him. I got the permit but didn't feel much safer. More important, I hated that it had come to this.

What started as a one-night refuge at Al and Marypat's house ended up lasting for a year. Days before I moved in, their second son, Sawyer, was born in their bedroom. The baby needed a lot of comforting, holding, walking. I helped out in the evenings. Sawyer and I were a good match. I craved his warmth and contact as much as he needed mine. I would hold his small body against me, rub his back, walk back and forth across the living room. I'd forget time, the stress of the day, the dizzy spiral of my life. The warm weight of Sawyer against me, the rise and fall of his breathing—this was medicine.

Eli, their older son, was a year and a half and fast on his feet. He would kick a ball in the yard with amazing accuracy and great delight. After a day at the office, I'd spend an hour in the yard, running after balls, kicking them back and forth with him, laughing at his antics. Becoming part of the family, and contributing, was an island of serenity. I found solace there, felt safe. I could almost fool myself into thinking that life was normal.

Late that spring, Blue Mountain Clinic in Missoula, two hundred miles west of Bozeman, was the target of an arson attack. It was a facility that provided all types of family medicine, family planning, and prenatal care, as well as abortions. Missoula was also where Michael Ross's letters came from. When I heard the news, I thought immediately of him. I sent copies of the letters I had received to the Missoula fire chief, including one that came just days after the arson. In that letter Ross suggested that my clinic would be the next to burn.

Nearly a week later the Missoula county attorney's office called me. They were appalled that no one had taken action against Michael Ross. "You've got to be kidding," they said. "This is a clear case of felony intimidation, no question. That's a federal offense." More than that, they were going to have him arrested and charged without delay.

I hung up and slumped onto my desk. Finally, someone who took this seriously, took my safety and well-being into account. As much as it would mean to be rid of this daily threat, it meant even more to have my concerns acknowledged.

Buffeted by this legal and personal turmoil, I found solace in holding tight to the memory of being supported by hundreds of thousands of people. In April of 1992, Flower Grandma, Mom, Sonja, and I, four generations of women, had attended the March for Women's Lives in Washington, DC. It was a glorious sunny day. Once again I was carried along in a wave of support and energy, surrounded by an ocean of commitment and goodwill. I marched on the front lines and was one of the speakers who addressed the crowd of a million pro-choice supporters.

As I spoke, I searched for Flower Grandma, seated at the front of the crowd.

"As long as you'll continue to stand up and support me," I said. "I'll continue to work. With you alongside I'll never have to feel alone." My words were for all the escorts, volunteers, staff, and political activists, but most of all, for Flower Grandma, for her childhood friend whose life was needlessly cut short, for all the women through time, everywhere, whose lives have been compromised. As I spoke, I could feel her strong, soft, loving hands holding mine. That promise, and the continued support of women's advocates, are what keep me strong to this day.

•

The first year in Montana went by in a blur. Michael Ross was arrested, tried, found guilty, and sent to federal prison. Even so, every day continued to be crowded with security guards, circuitous routes, tangled instructions, life on the run. I wore my shoulder harness with a .38 Special nearly all the time.

I took personal protection classes from a firearms instructor. I had grown up in a house full of guns, dozens of them. We had an indoor shooting range under the house, and all the siblings would compete after supper, routinely going through hundreds of rounds. We were all good shots and thoroughly versed in firearm safety.

There was never a loaded gun in the house, except in the shooting range. We were not even allowed toy guns. If you pointed your finger at another person and said "Bang!" you were in big trouble. Firearms were respected weapons, never toys.

The thought of having a loaded pistol on my body was completely foreign, and the feel of a gun under my clothes never got comfortable. It went against everything I had been taught. I kept having flashes of Dad and the lessons he hammered home. The instructor sensed my apprehension. He set out on a program to desensitize me. He had me shooting at cardboard human targets over and over. I shot from a standing position, sitting, lying across the hood of a car, kneeling beside a tree. He taught me to react quickly and accurately. Eventually, I could get my hands on the pistol, get it out of the holster, and be firing in seconds.

He told me I should have the pistol on me all the time, if only to get completely used to it. I always unloaded it when I came home to Marypat and Al's, but every day I wore it.

One of the first days I wore the gun, two acquaintances came by and asked if I would join them in a nearby café for a beer and a sandwich after work. I changed into jeans and a large, loose-knit sweater and went out the door, happy for the invitation. Midway through the meal I felt one of the loops on the sweater catch on the release of the holster. The pistol came loose and slipped under my arm. The heavy weapon flopped into the sweater fabric, started to slide toward my hip.

Just what I need, I thought. Way to make a great impression, guns falling out of my clothes. I shifted in my seat, squirmed to catch the gun against my hip, felt it slide further. Then, pretending I was arranging my napkin, I snatched the pistol and slipped it under my thigh. I sat on that gun for the rest of the evening. I couldn't even get up to use the bathroom.

When I told my father the story, he was not amused. To him, it was appalling. "I understand your need to carry a firearm," he said. "But you have to be responsible with it."

Actually, hardly anything was amusing for Dad anymore. His health had badly deteriorated. He'd lost weight and looked pale and drawn. Most of all, he had no energy. On good days it was all he could do to make a round trip from the house to the barn. We had very little idea what was going on. Tests and doctor visits hadn't turned up anything conclusive. I had made a decision to stay clear of his medical care and diagnoses. I wanted to be his daughter, not his doctor. With hindsight, I would realize that it was a bad decision, one that I'd feel debilitating guilt over.

I knew better than to tell Dad about the first time I actually drew the pistol, ready to protect myself. It happened on one of the many nights I worked late. When I finished, I really didn't want to sleep in the recliner, surrounded by work. I craved contact with a family.

The fact that Michael Ross was in custody had relieved my general sense of apprehension. There were a few local people who scared me, men who followed and harassed me, but they hadn't gotten to me the way Ross had with his incessant flow of letters.

I had become a regular topic of discussion in the local letters to the editor, the usual ugly rhetoric. There had been some wanted posters put up around town. At the same time, people regularly dropped by the office to express support. Several people left me their house keys and directions, no strings attached. If you need a refuge, just use it, they said.

It was almost midnight. I was nervous about leaving the building, but there were times when I couldn't stand any more of the clandestine sneaking around. The ability to leave and go home without an escort offered a thin thread of normalcy, a hint of sanity. The third floor was dark. I got into the elevator and pushed the button. At the first floor I was standing in the brightly lit elevator as the doors began to open. Suddenly, all the other lights on the first floor snapped off. I heard footsteps running in my direction.

Without thinking, I pulled the pistol and hugged the inside wall of the elevator. The man who charged in saw me and immediately threw his hands up, a terrified look on his face. I recognized him as an employee I'd seen around the building. I brought the gun down, stepped off the elevator, and hit the main floor light switches. Both of us were shaken up, but when he heard my explanation, he understood completely. After that night I resigned myself to calling Tom to escort me out of the building and get me home.

On the one-year anniversary of the clinic opening we held a party for local friends and supporters. Out of the blue, one of the women invited me to spend time at her ranch, a few miles from town. She said it was fairly isolated and had a long driveway. You could see anyone coming from a quarter mile away.

I'd been in Montana a year already but still hadn't spent any amount of time in the mountains. Comfortable as it was living with Marypat and Al, I couldn't stay forever, and an occasional night out of town sounded good.

The clinic had grown to the point that it was supporting itself. I stopped traveling to and from the Midwest each week. Sonja planned to spend the summer with me. The first night in the ranch house, I fell in love with it. So much of it was familiar—the outdoor sounds, the quiet, the nearby barn. It was rural and comfortable, so much like my childhood home in Wisconsin.

Before long, I moved into one of the houses on the ranch. I also bought a twenty-five-year-old Dodge camper van with a pop top. I named her Betty. On weekends when the weather was good, I'd load up Betty, hitch up the horse trailer, and head for another trailhead to explore. I'd ride one horse, pack the other with gear, and go high into the mountains. In summer, Sonja was with me. She was an accomplished camper and horsewoman in her own right.

Even when Sonja wasn't with me, we talked almost daily by phone. She told me about her classes and friends, her swim meets, what she was making for supper. In some ways we talked more than most mothers and daughters because we made such a point of staying connected across distance. There was a kind of safety offered by the telephone. We didn't have to face each other with more difficult topics, but had the buffer of the phone line. Strangely, I think we were more honest and revealing than we would have been living in the same house.

Randy was always reassuring. He helped Sonja with her homework, went to her swim meets, attended school conferences, never wavered in his day-to-day commitment. In spite of that, Randy and I continued to drift apart, each of us consumed with our own existence, a thousand miles from each other. More and more, our phone conversations stuck to the logistics of life and avoided the obvious—we were less and less of a couple. The very traits that were essential for my career—stubbornness, single-mindedness, independence, being firmly in control—were detrimental when it came to my marriage.

On the ranch in Montana, I could finally have my horses with me, go for early morning rides, hike along the ridge and fish in the creek, hear elk bugle in the fall. That country place was a spiritual sanctuary, a place of soothing refreshment, a place to center myself within the storm of life.

Always, though, above everything, it was the patients who brought me comfort. Many of them were caught up in personal turmoil and stress, but there is something fundamentally rewarding about connecting with a stranger in need, coming to grips with her situation, and acting in tangible ways to resolve problems. Each day brought a different set of stories, every one compelling and vivid—stories wrapped in life's ironies and intricacies. Every day brought with it some piece of amazement.

To All at Mountain Country Women's Clinic:

I really don't know how to thank all of you.
Each of you played an important role in
making a very scary, negative situation a
positive one that resulted in a second
chance for me. I spent a week of my life in a
trance of dread and hopelessness, full of
fear. However, after my first visit to your
clinic this feeling began to fade. Everybody
was honest, in all aspects. Never did I feel
isolated, pressured, or alone. I can now go
on with my life knowing I made the best
decision, and I plan on making it one hell
of a life!

Former Patient

— chapter nine

The day begins with the pager going off as I get out of the shower at six-fifteen AM. The answering service. I pull on my bathrobe while I call in. "It's a woman who says she has an emergency," the operator says. "I'll put her through."

All I hear at first is uncontrollable sobbing. Then a voice. "I'm pregnant! I have to talk to someone. I don't know what to do!" Words between hysterical sobs.

"Take a deep breath, and give yourself a second so we can talk. I'm sure things are going to be alright."

"But I'm pregnant!" she wails. "It's not alright! What am I going to do?"

"You tell me," I reply in a quiet voice. "Tell me what you are thinking."

"I'm thinking that I cannot stay pregnant! I have to have one of those abortions."

"Are you sure? There are a number of options you know. Have you thought about adoption?" I speak slowly and calmly, still dripping water all over the floor.

"No. No. No. I have to have one of those abortions. I can't be pregnant. How many days will it take?" she asks, fear creeping into her voice.

"Days? The procedure only takes a few minutes." I am once again amazed at the misinformation out there.

"But will I bleed a lot? Will I ever be able to have children again? Could I die?" the questions fire out in quick succession.

"Just a second. Take another deep breath, and let me ask you a few questions. Okay. Now, how overdue is your period?"

"Only a week," she sniffles.

"Good. In a pregnancy that early you are really safe having an abortion. You'd be in the clinic several hours, but most of that time is spent in counseling and recovery. The procedure actually takes only five minutes and is very safe. It is, in fact, much safer than going through a full term pregnancy and delivery. And as far as future fertility, there is absolutely no medical evidence that suggests uncomplicated first trimester abortions cause infertility or miscarriages in the future. You will be just fine.

"The most important thing is your personal choice. This has to be your choice, not someone else's." She has been quiet, listening. Her breathing slows. She's calmed down a notch.

"Can my husband come, too?"

"Of course he can. We encourage you to bring someone who will support you." There is a pause.

"Are you feeling better?"

"Yes, I guess," she replies, an obvious change in her voice.

We talk another five minutes. She tells me about having four kids at home, about her financial situation.

"Listen, if you are absolutely sure about this, you can call in after eight and make an appointment. Or come in, and we'll just talk about it. You are in no danger. We'll answer any questions you have and give you referrals for other options. This is entirely your choice. Okay?"

By the time I'm off the phone I'm already behind. No time for breakfast. I down a cup of coffee while I dress, strap on the pistol, grab the backpack with the ever-present camera and tape recorder in case I need to document something. I am not in the mood for the bulletproof vest and leave it behind. I go in streaks with the vest. It is such a solid reminder of the threats I get and the diligence I have to maintain. Oddly, the pistol in the shoulder harness has become a natural part of my existence, but the vest makes me feel more like a target.

I head out the door just as Tom drives up. We both routinely check the road as we drive out, looking for unfamiliar cars, parked cars with a person inside, pedestrians. If something looks out of place, I jot down the details in my notebook: license number, descriptions of vehicles or people. As we drive to the clinic, we check the cars behind us, watch down the alleys and cross streets. All this is automatic now, part of the way I think. We drive all around the clinic block, looking for anti-abortion bumper stickers, people standing on sidewalks who look out of place.

"Let's use the front door, Tom. We've gotten in the habit of always going in the back way."

He nods. "We might want to vary our arrival time, too. It's been pretty consistent lately. Maybe tomorrow I can pick you up ten minutes earlier."

Tom leads the way inside, always walks ahead. He is first in and out of the elevator. Everything is quiet. The clinic is dark, undisturbed.

I punch off the security system as I open up, and Tom goes with me through every room, opening doors, turning on lights, unlocking cabinets. I make a pot of coffee, look through the appointment book. There are days that I can tell will be abnormally hectic just by glancing at the appointments, but today doesn't look bad.

"Okay, Sue. See you tonight. Call if anything comes up," and Tom goes out. I lock the door behind him until another staff member shows up.

The first patient of the day is a fifty-seven-year-old woman who wants a routine checkup. She has been through menopause and hasn't had an exam in three years. We go through the usual lab work and a physical exam.

"I'm glad you are here," she says, and her voice trails off.

"There is something else, isn't there?" I ask. "What's on your mind?"

"Well, there is one thing," she says rather quietly, struggling to go on. "Sex has become painful lately. It's gotten so I'm not very interested anymore, and I wish I could do something about it."

I sit down, and we talk about the effects of menopause, some possible solutions. By the time she leaves she is visibly relieved. This one question is really why she came.

An abortion patient is just going in to the counseling room with one of the staff. Her lab work is finished, and I have a short break. I call two doctors about patients I've seen in the last few weeks. Both have been in for their follow-up exams; both are doing fine. I call another doctor about a recent patient who had an abnormal Pap smear. I think about calling home before Sonja goes to school, but realize it's already too late. Then I overhear the receptionist taking another call. Something in her voice makes me listen.

"I'm sorry, sir, but I can't give you that information," she says. "I can't answer that." A pause. "I'm sorry you feel that way." Her voice is increasingly firm. "I can't help you. I'll give the doctor your message." By the time she hangs up I'm standing next to her.

She points to an entry in the appointment book. "That was a man calling about this person right here. He said he's her uncle. He knows she's coming in, and he knows when her appointment is. He kept saying to tell the doctor if he kills that baby, he'll pay. He just kept saying, 'You better not kill that baby. That girl's too young.'"

The rest of the clinic staff have gathered by now, questioning, the level of anxiety rising. Then the phone rings again. The receptionist listens for several minutes, hangs up the phone, and turns to us. "That was the girl's aunt this time. She's on the way here. She said she forbids us to 'kill that baby.' She forbids us to even talk to the girl and says she is coming right now to stop us."

Everyone looks at me. "First of all, it's not their right to choose for her. It's her choice, and that's that."

"But they said they forbid it!"

"It's not theirs to forbid," I add firmly.

I walk away briskly, go into my office, and close the door. I need to gather my thoughts. My reaction was certain, but visceral. I need to get it together. This is my call, my challenge.

"I'm sorry I walked off," I say, when I return. "We need to be in control of this. If the patient comes in, she goes right to the back. I don't want her sitting in the waiting room. We'll do the lab and counseling in the back and not send her into the waiting room between times." Everyone is nodding in agreement.

"Okay. We need to call the police. Tell them we have a potential confrontation developing and that if we call for help it won't be just for a few hecklers out front. And erase her name from the appointment book."

There are several patients in the waiting room. I go out to talk with them. "There's a chance there will be some trouble with a patient's relative today. It has nothing to do with any of you, and it probably won't amount to anything, but if we ask you to move to another place, it will be for your safety. Please do as we ask, and do it quickly. And please, whatever happens, don't get involved."

"Okay, let's not let this distract us," I say to the staff. "No use worrying before anything happens. We have other patients to care for." As I head back through the office, I detour to a window overlooking the street. No protesters yet. Quiet outside.

Just then I hear the door open, and my instincts tell me it is the young woman in question. I get to the front just in time to hear her give the receptionist her name. I reach across the counter and touch her hand lightly. "Come on back with me," I say, "and bring your friend along." She and a girlfriend have arrived more than an hour early, having driven almost 150 miles. I bring the two of them into my office and close the door.

"We need to talk." I tell her briefly what has happened, see the weight of her dilemma settle on her. "Is your boyfriend with you?"

"No," she says. "He stayed home and went to work so everything would look normal. He works at a sawmill with my uncle. Somehow my uncle must have made him talk. This means I can't do it, doesn't it?" She is crestfallen.

"That is not at all what this means," I reassure her. "This is your decision and nobody else's. It's good you're here early for the appointment. But before anything, I need to know if you've thought through your decision, if you're completely sure about ending this pregnancy."

"Are you kidding? I can't be pregnant. I have a full scholarship to college starting this fall. There is no way. It would mean giving up everything. I'll have kids when I can take care of them."

Her demeanor reinforces what she says. She is unwavering, self-confident, mature. "Mark and I have talked it over a lot. This is what I have to do!"

"Do your parents know?"

She shakes her head.

"What would they say?"

"I thought about telling them. I know they would have been upset, but I think they'd probably support me. I just

— 135 —

didn't want to hurt them. Now my uncle has probably told them. Can he stop me? He is just such a fanatic about some things."

"No, he can't. He can't decide this, and we won't let him interfere."

"He's an awful man," she says. "He could hurt someone."

"Let us worry about him. You're our priority patient right now, and we need to get your counseling and lab work started. Perhaps we can get you out of here before they arrive, if they really are on their way. In any case, we'll keep you back here, out of sight."

The staff starts working on her lab tests. Another patient has finished her counseling and is ready for her abortion. I try hard to maintain an everything-is-normal manner. Before starting the procedure I make a call to a lawyer in town who, when I first opened the clinic, made a point of offering his services. I fill him in on what's happening. He promises to stay available, tells me to be careful. After I hang up, I readjust the shoulder harness on my pistol, feeling its heavy presence under my scrubs.

So much for an uneventful day, I think, as I go into the procedure room. All the way through that abortion I listen for the sound of the office door, for angry voices.

By the time the first patient is in recovery, we're ready to go. Her chart is straightforward. She has gone through the informed consent form and signed off. Her vital signs are perfect, and she has no medical history to worry about. I close the chart and enter the room where she is waiting for me.

"Okay," I start out, when I get inside. "Let's forget all about your uncle. He has nothing to do with this. Have you had all your questions answered? Do you understand the procedure? Have you had any other surgeries or any condition we should know about?"

Given the stress she is under, she is very articulate and very steady. We review things quickly but thoroughly. She shows no doubts.

"I'm going to step out now while you undress from the waist down. When you're undressed you can sit on the end of the table and cover with this drape."

I close the door and walk back to the window again. Still quiet outside. I check the waiting room, give the receptionist a squeeze on the arm before I go back.

"Before we start, I want to ask you again: Are you absolutely sure you want to have this abortion? Is there anyone pushing you or telling you to be here? Is this really your decision?"

She is sure.

She lies down for the ultrasound. "That's your uterus," I point to the screen. "Here's the fetal tissue. It looks normal for about five weeks gestation." There is a small sac attached to one side of the uterine wall.

"Now I'm going to do a regular pelvic exam. I'll touch your leg so you'll know where I am. I'm feeling inside for your cervix." At the same time I palpate her lower abdomen. "There is your uterus," I push down gently. "It feels really normal, maybe tipped back just a little. Is there any tenderness there?" I move my hand and press over her ovaries.

"Now we put these sterile drapes under you." I ready the instrument tray and sit at the end of the table. "I'll be using a speculum. It won't hurt, and it's all warmed up already. It just allows me to see your cervix and create a space to work through. If you have any questions at any time, please ask."

"I'm looking at your cervix now. Everything looks just fine. I'll clean the cervix and take a culture with a swab."

As I work, my assistant, a nurse, holds the bottle of lidocaine so I can draw it up into a syringe. "Most people don't feel these shots at all. If you feel anything, it will be a little pinch. First I numb the surface of the cervix. Now I can hold your cervix with an instrument that keeps everything steady while I put in two more injections. Tell me if you feel anything at all. There. That's that. Did you feel anything?"

She shakes her head.

"Now we'll let that numb up a minute. You take some big, deep breaths. Try and relax." My voice is a constant monotone. Even if there is nothing to say about the procedure, I talk about anything. The weather. How school is going. Where they work. How the drive was. Just keep talking with that soothing voice. I have changed into a new set of sterile gloves now and start explaining the next stage of the process, reinforcing what she has already heard in the counseling session. Always talking.

"These are the dilators." I show her the instruments. "When I use them, you'll feel a little tugging, but it won't be painful. I insert and then remove these gently, one at a time, in increasing size, until your cervix is dilated to about the diameter of a pencil." As I talk, I start the dilating. "When a woman delivers a baby, her cervix is dilated to ten centimeters. We're dilating your cervix to just seven millimeters, which is less than one centimeter. Keep your bottom muscles loose. But, please, if it does feel painful, let me know. I will stop and put in more pain meds. Now, another dilator. Take a deep breath in; hold it a few seconds. Now exhale, long and slow. Keep relaxing all your muscles. Good. One more now. Keep breathing." I find myself breathing along with her, as is the nurse.

"Any questions? Doing okay?" Always the same steady, soothing cadence to my voice.

"I'm fine," she says. My instruments clank softly on the tray.

"Okay, your cervix is dilated." As I say this, the nurse hands me a small, sterile tube attached to a device that creates a gentle suction. "This will feel really weird. That's the only way to describe it. It will be like a bubbling inside you, and you'll feel movement from the instruments, but very little pain. We suction for thirty to forty-five seconds." The machine always makes me think of an old refrigerator, that same deep hum.

When we finish, I rub her lower abdomen gently. "You may feel a strong deep cramp," I tell her. She nods emphatically. "That's good. It's your uterus contracting down, shrinking again. It's a good sign. Just keep breathing deep; relax."

I check the inside of her uterus with a curette, a small looped instrument, and finish with another ten seconds of suctioning. She handles it well, and soon I am picking things up, and the nurse is checking her blood pressure and pulse.

"It's over?" she asks. "Really, that's it? I'm not pregnant anymore? That isn't anything like what I heard it would be."

"Once in a while someone has a difficult abortion," I say. "But it is almost always someone with a fibroid growth or preexisting infection. Most are like yours."

While the nurse escorts her to the recovery room, I take the fetal tissue to the lab. Still no sign of trouble in the office. I remove the quarter-sized sac from the jar. It is filmy with placental tissue and some of the endometrium that normally sloughs off. All normal.

I always give patients the option of seeing the tissue if they want to, and this woman wants to see it. "That's all?" she says when I show it to her. She escapes into her own thoughts for a minute and looks at me with hesitation.

"What is it you're thinking?" I prod.

"How can it be that my uncle believes I am less important than that tiny bit of tissue you just took out of me?"

She isn't expecting me to respond. She is talking to herself, trying to put her world in order. I sit quietly with her for a few minutes.

We finally start talking about home care, birth control, and general recovery issues. Patients generally stay for at least thirty minutes so we can be sure they are stable. She wants to leave after just ten minutes, hoping to be gone before her uncle and aunt get there, if they really are coming. But I make her stay the full thirty minutes. Taking short cuts with her health is not an option. In the meantime I leave her with the nurse and excuse myself to go see another patient.

Finally, we are escorting her out of the clinic with her girlfriend, after having checked the corridor and elevator for signs of her relatives. I wrap my arms around her briefly as she passes through the door. The waiting room is tense. Then I let her go. The two of them hurry out of sight.

All of the staff is lined up at the window overlooking the parking lot. I hear one of them muttering urgently, "C'mon, girl, get out of here!" Finally we see them, moving quickly, getting into the van they arrived in. All of us are half-dancing with tension at the window. Finally they turn out of the parking lot, down a side street—the blinker flashes—gone.

"Yes." I breathe. And we all turn back, grinning our relief. There are so many women who leave the office to return to their uncertain receptions, their uncertain futures. If only we could fast-forward for a glimpse to better prepare ourselves.

We are behind schedule now, and the weight of the pistol drags on my consciousness. We aren't through this yet, I remind myself. And as I ready myself for the next patient, I hear a man's voice at the reception desk, an ugly voice.

"Where's that doctor?"

No time to think, just react. I suppress the momentary urge to hide, forcing myself out front.

"Where's that doctor?" he repeats, and I can see him leaning aggressively over the counter. A heavy man, tiny sharp eyes, thick gnarled hands out in front of him.

"I'm right here," I announce. "What can I do for you?"

"YOU?" he is thrown off. He expected a man. Now I see a woman behind him, a tall, skinny figure with gray hair. She is craning for a look at me.

"Yes. What can we do for you?"

"We know Grace is here. You can't kill that baby. We're here to take her home."

The other people in the waiting room are all ears and eyes, the tension palpable. One gathers her coat in her lap. They glance at each other.

"We have no one by that name here. There is no one by that name in the appointment book at this time. You have no business disrupting this office!"

"Office!" he sneers. "This—this slaughterhouse? You're a killer! You call yourself a doctor?"

"That's enough!" the strength in my voice comes from somewhere I can't fathom, overriding the fear, pushing aside the ugliness emanating from this man. Then I catch a glimpse of a young man standing just inside the door. He is shifting nervously, looking everywhere but at me. The boyfriend, I think. "That's enough! There is no one here for you, and you have no business with my office. You'll have to leave."

"We know she is coming!" he tries to look around me to the back rooms. "You're not killing that little baby!"

"You'll have to leave. Now!" I come around to herd them out, thinking about the pistol as I approach, watching the man and woman. "There are chairs by the elevator. If you must waste your time, I can't stop you from sitting out there."

They are backing up. The woman's eyes are burning with anger. The boyfriend is already out, more than willing to leave. "You'll have some answering to do!" I hear the uncle say to him in the corridor. On their way to the chairs in the hall-way the man turns to me again, shaking his fist. "And you'll answer, too, you doctor!" he spits the words. "You'll answer!"

I shut the door on them, lean against it briefly, and try hard to make my smile reassuring for the waiting-room audience.

"Sue," the receptionist interrupts. "Sonja's on the phone."

I step into my office, pause, take a big breath. "Hi Begonia!" I use my Happy Mom voice. We chat briefly before Sonja springs the real reason for her call.

"Mom, a week from Friday is the parent/student swim meet. You know, parents against the swim team." Silence.

"Mom," she brings me back. "Randy doesn't swim. Can you come home?"

I take another breath, try to get everything back in perspective. "I'll do my best, sweetie."

Then the call is cut short when one of the counselors knocks on the door.

"Can you come help for a minute? This one needs some comforting," she whispers. I sigh, say good-bye to Sonja, gather myself, try to push the people in the hallway out of my mind. But I'm still flushed from the confrontation.

When I enter with the counselor, I recognize the patient. I saw her arrive earlier. She edged in through the door as if she were afraid it would slam and lock behind her. College age, jumpy, from a rural area, I expect. She confirmed her appointment without approaching the counter, sat right next to the door, never took her coat off. I see that even in the counseling room she is balanced on the edge of her chair, flinches when I close the door.

"Hi," I say. "I'm the doctor." She nods, gulps, looks away.

"Is everything alright?" She nods too emphatically.

"Have you been somewhere else for a pregnancy test?"

She looks surprised, makes eye contact for the first time.

"Was it the clinic that advertises abortion information in the paper?"

"How did you know?"

"You act the way most people do after they've been there," I tell her. "We aren't the same kind of place. And I doubt we're anything like what they told you there." I have her attention now.

"I thought I'd be able to get an abortion there," she admits. "They looked like nurses and doctors with their white coats. They told me they were giving me a pregnancy test and put me in a room for two hours. There was a television playing an awful video in there. I couldn't leave."

I sit in front of her and give her all my attention, encouraging her to keep talking.

"When they told me my test was positive, they started saying there was a good chance I'd bleed to death from an abortion. That I ought to consider keeping the baby. That I'd regret this the rest of my life."

"And," I say as I hold her attention, "they told you you'd probably never have children after having an abortion, right?"

"How did you know?"

"And they told you there was a good chance you'd die, right? And that I am not a real doctor? That if you came here you could get AIDS from other patients?" She is open-mouthed, nodding.

"First of all, you are completely free to leave any time you want. We will answer any questions you have. This isn't something we do to you. You can decide to have this done. If you want to talk about adoption, about social services available for mothers without money, about prenatal care, about any of that stuff, that's fine. We have lots of information available on all the options, including accurate information about abortion."

She is visibly relaxed, although she still looks guardedly back and forth between us, like we might be tricking her yet.

"They told me you have knives and scissors here. That you cut up babies and throw them in the garbage!"

"There are no knives, no scissors, no scalpels. If patients want to see the embryonic tissue, we give them that option. Most women are actually quite relieved when they see it. And we take great care disposing of it in a respectful, appropriate, legal manner.

"The very last thing we want is for you to make a bad decision. You got some wrong information. Let me just tell you this. There is a greater chance you'll die in a car wreck on your way to the office than there is of a serious complication with an abortion." She is listening intently now, looking at me closely.

"We use gentle dilation and suction." I show her some tubing, dilators, and a speculum. "There is no cutting, no intense pain. Those gruesome pictures they showed you have nothing to do with the reality of what we do here.

"The most important thing is that you make the right decision. And if you want to find out about my credentials, you should call the medical board. I'll give you the number."

"That's okay," she says. "I believe you."

"Good. Now we've got that behind us. Why don't you start the counseling over again? Can we do that?" I get up to go.

The amazing thing, I think as I close the door, is that they still come. After hearing all that terrible propaganda and lies

and being shown the inaccurate pictures by the places calling themselves some version of a pregnancy counseling center, they still come. They are desperate to end an unwanted
pregnancy.

Back in my office I collect myself for a minute. I'm the
one who needs a little settling before I go on. And it's barely
lunchtime. I realize how hungry I am and pick up the phone
to order some sandwiches for the staff. As I order, I stroll to
the window. Half a dozen protesters parade slowly along,
holding their signs, watching people come and go. All of
them are regulars; four out of the six are men.

Since a recent court injunction they have been forced to
stay on the sidewalk below and are banned from coming inside the building or accosting patients in the parking lot.
"Sidewalk counseling" they call their harassment. "If you saw
a murder in progress, wouldn't you try to stop it?" one of
them asked the judge at the hearing. Absently I check the lot
for strangers, anything out of place.

I see the morning patient's aunt appear around the corner
of the building. She is doing her own checking, no doubt
looking for her niece's car. She looks perplexed, angry, impatient. She stops and watches the protesters for a second. I
wonder if she'll go over to them, but she continues on
through the lot, then comes back inside.

There are two more procedures before I get a chance to
eat the soggy sandwich that has been waiting on my desk. I
see a phone message from the British television people who
have been after me for an interview about violence against
abortion providers in America. I remember to call the lawyer

from the Center for Reproductive Law and Policy who is working on getting the FDA to approve a version of the morning-after pill. So much to do.

Another message under a file folder. This one from a local man who has offered his mountain cabin for a staff retreat if we ever need a break. How about right now? I think to myself, ruefully. Right now would be great! I smile, visions of ski trails, a wood stove pulsing heat, silent stars in a black sky. Enticing as the scene is, the gesture of support is better still. But here and now we are behind schedule, and the young, frightened patient is ready. I glance over her chart before I go in.

"How are you doing now?" I ask her, as I pull up the stool to talk before we begin.

"Better," she says, and she looks better, even a little sheepish.

Within ten minutes we have completed the abortion without incident, and I head up to the front desk. The receptionist looks exhausted as she lifts her head and gestures toward the waiting room. The young boyfriend is sitting there, head down, looking at his hands.

"He came in a few minutes ago. He looked so sad when he asked if he could sit in here. He said he couldn't stand it out there with them. I couldn't say no."

I nod. An overwhelming urge to go to him wells up in me. I want to go sit by him, whisper that she's been here, that she's fine, that everything is okay. He'll know soon enough, but that anguish on his face is almost unbearable, when I could remove it so easily.

A tap on my shoulder. "I think we have a fake one," the counselor says. "Maybe we should team up on her a little." I give the waiting room one more glance, hoping to catch the young man's eye, hoping I can say what I want to say with a look, but he doesn't raise his head.

"Her urine sample wasn't even warm," the counselor tells me. "Of course it was positive, but she doesn't seem right. She keeps asking questions about the clinic hours, what days you are here, stuff like that." We start to go in, but the counselor stops me again. "I think she's got a tape recorder going."

When we both enter the room, the patient fidgets nervously, gives us a forced smile.

"Hi. I'm Dr. Wicklund," I say, and I extend my hand. She takes it gingerly, quickly.

"Tell me about yourself," I prompt her.

"Well," she says, brightly. "I'm twenty years old. I already have three children, and I've been on welfare for a while. Now I'm pregnant. Do you think I should have an abortion?"

"What I think isn't very important." I smile back. "It's what you think that matters. Have you thought about your options? Have you considered adoption?"

"Oh, I don't know about that," she says, looking back and forth between us. "I think I should have an abortion, don't you?" There is no emotion coming from her, not even the forced control some patients impose on themselves. She talks as if she's playing a game. Likely, she is.

"If you have to ask us what we think, you aren't clear enough about it." I pull an informed consent sheet from a nearby drawer and hand it to her. "Please read through this.

It will give you some information about the risks and alternatives and the procedure." She barely glances at it. "We'll give you some pamphlets about adoption and the social service agencies to contact. You need to gather more information and not ask someone else to make this decision for you. The counselor will show you out."

She looks momentarily flustered, as if she is scrambling mentally for some way to stay, then gives in and starts putting on her coat. She leaves the informed consent sheet behind and refuses the additional information we try to give her.

"Could have been worse," I shrug, "but it's still a waste of time."

At least she wasn't one of the disruptive ones. Some of them park themselves in the waiting room and start ranting. "I don't know," they fret. "I don't know if I want to kill my baby. Do you want to kill your baby?" They turn to the patient next to them, wringing their hands. "I don't know if I want to kill mine."

If you don't get control of those in a hurry, they can have the whole clinic in an uproar.

The next patient needs a routine yearly exam, and I need the basic, unemotional interaction to center myself again. We chat about her work, the prospects for a good ski year, general banalities. She is perfectly sound, absolutely healthy, and I find myself grateful to this woman for her mundane normality.

The people are still sitting in the hall, their presence brooding outside like dead air before a storm. They assume either that we have their niece hidden in a back closet or that she is yet to come. At least they've been quiet since the first outburst.

What would we have done if they had trapped her here? Police escort, probably. And what will she face at home now? The uncle's angry face is fresh in my mind.

Two more abortion patients cycle through the lengthy process. They tell their stories, talk everything through with a counselor. Each of them undresses, entrusts herself to my hands, listens intently to my droning voice all the way through the procedure. Most wear a look of relief and gratitude as they leave. There is much that has become standard and routine over the years. Things I have done thousands of times. Yet each patient is unique. Each has her own set of fears, her own hopes and dreams and emotions. Every woman has personal reasons behind her choice that are hers alone. Nothing is routine about any of this for them. And for the life of me, I couldn't describe the common reasons for abortions, couldn't sketch the typical patient.

The work day won't let go easily. The final patient is one of the cases I dread. She is unsure of her last normal menstrual period, and as soon as I begin the ultrasound I know she is into the second trimester of the pregnancy. The measurements put her pregnancy at seventeen weeks, well past my usual cutoff date.

"Why don't you sit up?" I say, gently. "Let's talk a minute."

She is concerned, already on the verge of tears. "What's wrong?"

"It appears that you are further along in the pregnancy than you may have thought. We have a lot to talk about, and you have more to think about."

She is starting to cry, and I move in to hold her for a brief second.

"Why don't you get dressed? We can't talk properly when you're half naked. I'll step out, and we'll go to my office."

"This means you won't do it?" she says when we are seated. "You can't do it? What am I going to do now?" She is crying in earnest. I go and hold her again, say nothing.

"I spent all my money on the bus to get here. How can I get another day off? Where will the money come from? I thought it would be over today, that I wouldn't be pregnant after today."

"I know. I know," I soothe her. "You had no idea."

She looks at me, imploring. She is young, alone, devastated. She has traveled almost three hundred miles by herself, has gathered all her resources for this.

"I can't do an abortion for you. I'm really sorry. I have made a personal decision not to do abortions after fourteen weeks.

"There are places that will help you if you still decide to have an abortion," I tell her. "We'll give you the numbers. If you want us to help you contact them, we can call from our office today. Even if you just want to talk things over, call the 800 number any time. I'm really sorry."

It is half an hour before she is in shape to leave. We refund her money; one of the staff gives her a ride to the bus station. Our patient day is over, but I can't turn it off like that, not with the memory of the morning patient. Not thinking about this last young girl on her seven-hour bus ride home. Home to what? Will someone be there to hold her?

The staff is tidying up, locking doors, making sure the day's paperwork is complete. I heave an end-of-the-day sigh and pitch in to help. The young man in the waiting room leaves again, quietly, still downcast.

Tom arrives to escort us all out.

"Oh wait," I interrupt. "We need to look at the schedule for the end of next week. I think Betty and I will be making the drive back to the Midwest for a few days. Turns out I have to compete in a swim meet!"

In the hallway we confront the suspicious glare of the aunt and uncle. "We're closing up now," I announce. "You can sit here a little longer if you want, but the building closes soon." They say nothing as we troop past.

Tired and preoccupied as I am, I can't afford to give in to it. I read every stranger's face in the corridors of the building, study the cars in the lot. We drive a new route home.

"More bad letters in today's mail?" Tom asks.

"One. But I didn't have time to dwell on it. I hardly read it—just put it in the file."

We idle in the driveway and make arrangements for the next morning. Then I'm done.

But I'm never really done. When I go to a movie later that evening, I see one former patient in the ticket line, another in the lobby. We make eye contact. One of them says "hi" in a whisper. I let them lead these interactions. Sometimes they give me an update on their lives; sometimes they ignore me; most often there is that moment of strong eye contact, a brief nod, our confidential bond, then on with our lives.

Very late at night the phone rings—1:30 blinks at me from the clock as I grope for the phone. "Dr. Wicklund? There is a woman on the line. She says it's an emergency." It is never over, I think, waiting to be put through, waiting to find out what kind of an emergency it might be. Then I realize that the day did end and that this is another, new day.

A 2006 Congressional investigation of federally funded "Crisis Pregnancy Centers" (CPCs) found that CPCs routinely misinform clients about health risks associated with abortions. CPCs are often affiliated with anti-choice organizations and have received more than thirty million federal dollars between 2001 and 2005. Of twenty-three CPCs investigated, twenty provided false or misleading information unsupported by scientific evidence. These CPCs claimed that there is a link between abortion and breast cancer, that abortion harms a woman's future fertility, and that abortion increases the risk of severe mental health problems. The Congressional report found that CPCs are engaging in an "inappropriate public health practice."

chapter ten

I fired up Betty at five AM on a Thursday, aiming for the starting blocks at the Cambridge High School pool a thousand miles away. I had twenty hours. I figured that if everything went smoothly, Betty could manage a fifty-mile-an-hour average, which would put me there on Friday afternoon with about an hour to spare. Betty and I wheeled into the parking lot with more like ten minutes of cushion.

Sonja was delighted. Her hug just about erased the road fatigue, and before I was ready, I was suited up and aligned with the rest of the sacrificial parents waiting for the start pistol. That the parents lost was a foregone conclusion. That I was there for Sonja was the triumph. Randy sat poolside, cheering for both of us.

Within days I was back on the same highway, driving into the sunset. I often drive without music or news on. I let the land flow past, the miles accumulate in my wake, and my thoughts roam. This is when I do some of my best thinking, sorting things out, and occasionally, stumble across a revelation. The warmth of my visit with Sonja and Randy faded in the distance. North Dakota spread ahead for hundreds of miles. My thoughts centered more and more on the many obstacles that get in the way of my direct interaction with patients, layers and layers of obstacles.

Legal and political distractions are a constant, energy-sapping aspect of my medical life. Right from the start of my career, and on an almost daily basis, I have been interrupted, distracted, and sometimes prevented from going about my work by legal skirmishing and political meddling in patients' lives.

A significant part of my work routine is tied up with phone calls to lawyers, appearances in court, and strategy sessions devoted to interpreting laws and coping with the latest challenge. Some of it is intensely personal and threatening, like testifying against letter-writer Michael Ross and even having to read his letters out loud to the jury. Much of it is so petty and ridiculous that it would be comical if it weren't such a nuisance and if it didn't have the effect of making the choice to end a pregnancy so fraught with roadblocks.

Protesters routinely take pictures of patients coming to a clinic, for example. Once, a friend of mine was visiting and decided to go outside and see how the protesters felt about her taking their pictures. The protesters called the police and the newspaper. The next day the local paper ran a story featuring the mystery woman taking pictures outside the clinic. Of course, the story never mentioned the picture-taking habit of the protesters.

While I worked in the Fargo clinic, protesters blatantly defied a court injunction banning them from being on the sidewalk in front of the doors. Once, out of frustration, the director turned on sprinklers to spray the walk. The protesters had the gall to call the police and report us. Worse yet, the police had the gall to cite us. A small thing, but unbelievably distracting and maddening.

Anti-choice politicians have enlisted in the battle. Laws and restrictive amendments are constantly being introduced. When a bill's passage looks problematic, it gets attached at the last minute to a broader measure. The legislation may be too vital to delay, so it will pass, saddling women and clinics with the ramifications. In recent years, state and federal politicians and judges have become increasingly brazen in their efforts to outlaw abortions altogether, subpoena clinics for their records, or place restrictions on clinics and patients. The Wisconsin legislature came very close to passing a law that would have banned the University of Wisconsin Student Health Care system from discussing anything about abortion with their students seeking information on pregnancy options. Even passing on phone numbers or names of abortion providers would have been illegal.

During the summer of 2006, Congress considered several draconian measures under the headings of the Child Interstate Abortion Notification Act (CIANA) and the Child Custody Protection Act (CCPA). Among other things, these proposals would make it illegal for someone other than a parent or legal guardian to transport an abortion patient across a state line. A grandmother, boyfriend, clergy, or older sibling would be risking arrest by doing so. In addition, the patient would have to satisfy regulations such as parental notification or mandatory waiting periods for both her state of residence and the state where the procedure is performed. If the patient wanted to seek a judicial bypass, she would have to do so in both states.

On a local level, anti-choice candidates have quietly become the majority on many school boards and county commissions, where they work to pass policies outlawing sex education in schools or declaring abortions illegal in their jurisdiction.

Some of the political maneuvering sounds innocuous or even positive. Of course parents should know about a daughter's pregnancy decision. Who would object to that? But what if that pregnancy is the result of incest, or the family has a history of domestic abuse? It also seems reasonable to consider a choice as weighty as abortion for at least a day. The fact is that the notification process burdens women with logistical, professional, and financial difficulties that in some cases make the abortion impossible.

No other medical procedure is shackled by such restrictions. Tubal ligation, vasectomy, and even open-heart surgery rely only on the discretion of a physician in consultation with his or her patient.

Much of the debate is couched in misleading and untrue statements. Embryonic tissue is referred to as an "unborn child." Breast cancer, infertility, and mental illness are commonly, and incorrectly, associated with abortions. It isn't uncommon for me to have to disabuse patients of the notion that they will be "scraped with a razor" during the abortion procedure.

The hyperbole can emanate from the highest levels of government. In July 2006 President Bush's press secretary replied that the president "doesn't condone murder" when he was asked why Bush would not support embryonic stem-cell research using frozen, unclaimed embryos.

The result of the pitched, moralistic battle is that abortion services have become marginalized within the medical community. Insurance policies often won't cover abortion services, although they routinely fund Viagra and similar drugs. Medical students are sent literature from anti-choice groups warning them to avoid training in abortion protocol. Many private medical practices forbid their partners to perform abortions. In the end, less than 10 percent of all abortions are performed in hospitals or in private physician's offices.

All that aside, the logistics alone make an abortion tenuous. I had a patient once who lived on an Indian reservation in northern Montana. When I examined her, I found scarring and cuts on her cervix. She had tried repeatedly to self-abort because she had no money and no vehicle, and the nearest clinic was a three-hundred-mile trip. Her aunt found out about her condition, scraped together funds, borrowed a dilapidated vehicle, and brought her to my clinic.

Many clinics are only open one day a week or several days a month. They get booked up weeks in advance. People may have to travel four hundred miles by car. They miss work, have to borrow money. By the time they are able to put together the resources to accomplish an abortion, the pregnancy is usually several months along.

Frivolous malpractice suits or assault charges brought against escorts are almost always overturned. Judges scold the plaintiffs for wasting court resources. But that isn't what the public remembers. The media reports the slanderous charges, blares them in headlines. That's what lodges in the public mind. By the time charges are dropped, years later and after significant expense, it is stale news buried in the back pages.

The choice community has its share of triumphs in the war, but they hardly ever feel triumphant. Pledge-A-Picketer campaigns raise money through local citizens pledging money for each picketer who appears before a clinic. The money is set aside for indigent women. At the end of every month a newspaper ad thanks the picketers for raising so much money and helping needy women get abortions. It doesn't take long for the picketers to evaporate.

During the summer of 1991, in Appleton, Wisconsin, Operation Rescue waged a massive and lengthy sit-in at a clinic. They chained themselves together in front of the doors, chanting, "Mommy, don't kill me!" and pounding on the walls. Some protesters superglued their hands to the front doors. Court costs sapped the clinic budget to the point that staff could barely be paid. Local politicians took sides against abortion or remained silent.

Desperate, clinic owner Maggie Cage ran a full-page newspaper ad.

Where are you? Where are all the people we've helped over the years? We need you now. When you needed us we were there. We held your hand and supported you. We see you in restaurants and at the grocery store, at PTA meetings and softball games. You are the business people, the school officials, the politicians, the voters. We kept you safe. We held your secrets. But now we need help. Where are you?

The outpouring of support was overwhelming. Women wrote apologetic letters chastising themselves for being apathetic. They vowed to fight for the clinic. Financial donations revitalized the budget. The pro-choice community was revived.

The triumphs, reassuring as they are, have a bittersweet taste. Why should the fight be necessary in the first place?

The time and resources squandered fighting the battle could be used to help women and provide more complete reproductive health care. And the bottom line? How many women, people who never appear in any statistical analysis, have been denied their fundamental, legal right to control their destinies because of legal restrictions or impossible circumstances imposed by the anti-choice onslaught?

●

I was walking from the lab to the front waiting room when I was stopped by one of the counselors. She had just finished "pre-court counseling" with a seventeen-year-old and wanted to talk to me.

"She is everything we want our daughters to be," she said. "Top of her class, plays volleyball on the varsity, has college plans for the fall. She even teaches Sunday school. But she is really torn up about telling her parents. She had a positive pregnancy test nearly six weeks ago and knew immediately that she wanted to end the pregnancy."

"It sounds like she comes from a solid family," I said. "Why can't she talk to her parents?"

"Her older sister had a baby out of wedlock two years ago. Her parents were outraged, took away all financial support, and told her that the only thing worse would have been to have an abortion. The sister moved away and is living a rough life as a single mom. This girl isn't ready to be a mother. She doesn't feel like she can confide in her parents. She's decided to go for a judicial bypass."

"What's your concern then?" I asked.

"Her periods have been irregular. She and her boyfriend used condoms, but she still got pregnant. I'm concerned about how far along she is, and how long the court bypass procedure might take."

"Okay, let's do an ultrasound and find out." I started toward the counseling room.

"Hello, Carol," I said to the young woman. "I'm the doctor here today, and I've been hearing about your situation. How are you doing?"

"I just wish I could be done with this," she sighed. "I've been thinking about this for more than a month, and I'm positive about my decision."

"I know, but we have to follow the law, whether we agree with it or not. According to the law, you either have to notify both parents about your abortion, or you have to go through the courts to get a judge's permission."

We talked more about her life, her college prospects, her sister's plight. Then I suggested the ultrasound so that we could know precisely what time frame we were working with.

"I have to tell you," I said. "We only perform first trimester abortions at this clinic. If you're farther along by the time you get the court's permission, you'll have to go somewhere else, spend a good deal more money, and have a more involved procedure."

She nodded.

As soon as I saw the ultrasound image, I knew we were close to the cutoff. She was twelve weeks along. We had one week to complete the court requirement and schedule an abortion.

Carol left with the information she needed to make her court appointment, and we scheduled her in to an already busy day, a week later.

Four days later she called the clinic in tears. "The judge cancelled my court case because of a family emergency," she said. "By the time he comes back, it'll be too late!"

In this case, the clinic manager stepped in and called a neighboring county to arrange a court appearance. As it turned out, Carol was able to get her permission from the court and finally go through the procedure.

Afterwards, I visited her in the recovery room. She was sobbing.

"Carol," I said, putting my hand on her arm, "Are you cramping?"

"No, no, not at all," she wiped her face, struggled to compose herself.

"Do you feel like you made the wrong decision?" I held my breath.

"Absolutely not," she said. "The problem is that I've missed two days of school last week and three days this week. I'm way behind on homework, and I know the school will let my parents know that I've been gone. I'll have to tell them something. I just don't know what."

"Wouldn't it be better to just tell them the truth?" I asked.

"Oh NO!" she said, shrinking away. "After what happened to my sister? Are you kidding? I could never do that."

Without the parental consent law, Carol would have had her abortion a month earlier, missing one day of school. For young women with families they can talk to, the law is unnecessary, even insulting. In thirty-four states, however, for women like Carol, parental notification regulations only worsen an already tenuous and stressful time and perhaps complicate their lives to the point that an abortion becomes impossible.

•

Twenty-eight states mandate specific counseling language to insure that patients give their "informed consent" before an abortion procedure. Twenty-four states also require a waiting period, usually twenty-four hours, between that counseling and an abortion.

Informed consent provisions specify that the doctor who will perform the abortion, or, in some cases, an agent of that doctor, has to contact the patient either face-to-face or by telephone and inform them on a variety of issues identified by politicians who have little or no knowledge of the actual procedure.

Some states require that a specific script be read to the patient. The text is often laden with hyperbole and emotionally charged language, referring to an embryo as an unborn child, for instance. The required information can include inaccurate references to fetal pain, a reminder that the father will be required to provide child support, and an encouragement to review materials on other options provided on a state-sponsored website. A thorough discussion of risks associated with the procedure is also mandated by law.

After that, the patient has to take twenty-four hours to think about her decision. Only then can she legally have an abortion. The penalties for not following these laws range from significant fines to prison sentences.

I spend many hours in the evenings and early mornings calling patients to provide them the information mandated by law so that they can avoid an additional trip to the clinic and absences from school or work. Putting all the information into context and explaining the bigger picture take a tremendous amount of time.

If I tell a woman that she could die from the abortion procedure and leave it at that, it scares the bejesus out of her. If, however, I explain that there is a higher risk of complications from wisdom tooth extraction, it puts the statement into perspective.

It isn't uncommon to play phone tag or fall prey to unforeseen problems that cause us to miss our phone session. Those patients may lose their appointments altogether or have to delay their procedures because we can't connect.

Sunday night. Judy B. is on my call list for 8:20. She has an appointment on Wednesday. I try to call, but the number I've been given is incorrect. Judy waits by the phone but never hears from me. Trivial error. Unintentional, but with huge consequences.

On Monday she calls the clinic to reschedule the call, and I get the correct number. There is still time. When I call on Tuesday morning, a man answers the phone. "Judy had to go to the hospital with our three-year-old. I'm home with the other four kids. Can you call on her cell phone?" he asks.

"Of course I can," I say, but I try three times and only get her voice mail.

The next morning Judy arrives for her appointment. We can't do it because she has failed to comply with the law.

"I HAVE to do this today. Please!" Judy says. "Today is my only day off for the next two weeks. I'll get fired if I miss another day."

"I am so sorry," I say. "The law is absolute. We really can't do it."

Reluctantly she reschedules. We take care of the informed consent process right there. She leaves in tears.

Several days later, Judy is finally able to have her abortion. She is angry and, as she predicted, has lost her job.

•

Ultimately, much of the abortion war is waged in the courtroom. From county courts to the Supreme Court, cases are in constant flux, susceptible to the political tenor of the moment, changes in judicial makeup, and social pressure exerted by politicians and advocacy groups.

Roe v. Wade gets all the attention, but off the radar, innocuous-seeming legal wrangling can change the landscape for clinics and patients in dramatic, profound ways.

In 1998 the courts found in favor of NOW and the National Women's Health Organization, which operates eight clinics in the United States, citing the Racketeer Influenced and Corrupt Organizations (RICO) Act to prevent organized groups from crossing state lines to participate in activities that have the effect of hindering commerce. Operation Rescue and other groups routinely traveled across state lines, organized protests, and hindered the conduct of clinics.

Operation Rescue faced heavy fines, and the decision had a chilling effect on their ability to continue harassing clinics. They were essentially shut down after the court decision and a period of relative peace ensued.

In 2006 the U.S. Supreme Court revisited the case and overturned the decision. As a direct result, Operation Rescue reorganized under the banner Operation Save America and undertook a massive onslaught against the lone clinic left in Mississippi. Their express goal was shutting down the Jackson clinic.

Operation Save America's leader, Reverend "Flip" Benham, presided over a burning of the Quran during one gathering. When asked what the Quran had to do with abortions, Benham stated that they were "different manifestations covering the same fist, the fist of the devil."

Protesters verbally abused patients coming and going from the clinic and blatantly ignored the limitations placed on them by city ordinance. Benham said that the clinic, along with his other targets, which included Millsaps College, a high school, the Jackson police department, and the local newspaper, represented "the gates of hell."

In April 2007 the Supreme Court upheld the Partial-Birth Abortion Ban, reversing an earlier Supreme Court decision. It was the first time that the high court has mandated what a physician can or can't do with a patient and opened the door for more severe restrictions on abortion rights. This decision makes it illegal for doctors to perform what may be the safest medical procedure for women having second-trimester abortions. Less than five percent of all abortions fall into this category. They are often performed to save the life of the mother, in response to severe fetal anomalies, or to end a pregnancy that has been shown to be incompatible with life.

•

The legal and political furor focuses on the rights of embryonic tissue, not on the rights of women and young girls. All the attention is lavished on "the unborn." The restrictions are cynically referred to as a "woman's right to know," when, in fact, they do everything to prevent women from exercising their legal options. If the right to know is sacrosanct, why is our foreign and domestic funding muzzled by gag laws that prevent physicians from even discussing legal health care measures available to women?

In clinics, though, it is women we are dealing with, and girls. Where is the public outcry in defense of victims of domestic abuse, rape, and incest? Who is pursuing absent fathers who walk away from responsibility? Where are the protections of confidentiality for our patients?

Every day people come through our doors coping with real-life dilemmas and traumas. I often wonder if it were men who got pregnant, men who faced these wrenching personal difficulties, whether abortion would even be on the political radar. Would men be expected to compromise their futures, give up the prospect of college, lose professional opportunities, sacrifice their ambitions . . . to fatherhood? I suspect not.

In some cases, our patients face real danger. It is our job, our duty, to serve and help them. It is up to us to recognize their plight and to provide resources. No politicians or laws help us in that process. We have to rely instead on common sense, experience, and intuition. That duty requires the ability to ferret out the shape of a situation and intervene if necessary.

•

"This one's really young," the nurse warns me one day in clinic. "Her father is here, and he's awfully protective."

I look at her form. Fourteen, it says. But when I see her, she looks twelve. Twelve and terrified.

"Come on back," I beckon her down the hall. Her father follows her. A small man, unshaven, with nervous hands.

"I just want what's best for my girl," he says, looking right at me over his daughter's head.

"Is your wife here?"

He shakes his head. "We don't want to bother her mama with this. She wouldn't take it well.

"My girl's made a mistake, and we want to do what's best."

The girl stands quietly, head down.

"It will be an hour or so before your daughter's finished," I tell him. "You can wait up front."

"I can comfort her," he pleads. "I want to be with my girl."

"She'll be fine. Please."

He backs away, looks hard at his daughter, who won't look back.

I take her thin arm with my hand and lead her into the procedure room.

"Let's talk for a minute," I say.

She sits straight-backed, hands clasped in her lap. She looks cold.

I ask her general questions about her home, her family, how the drive was, what she likes about school. Her answers are small whispers.

I go on to tell her about the abortion, what we will be doing.

"Are you sure you want to do this?" I ask, finally coming to the point.

"I have to," she talks to the floor.

"Why?"

No response.

"Do you want to be pregnant?"

She shakes her head.

"Do you want an abortion?"

Another shake.

Alarm bells had started going off when I saw her interaction with her father. It was time to figure some things out.

"Do you have a boyfriend?"

Silence.

"Did a boyfriend get you pregnant?"

Nothing. I can see her shivering.

I move closer. I want to hold her, make her warm and unafraid, but I know that's the wrong move. "Listen," I say, gently. "Sometimes things happen that aren't easy to talk about. I need to know how you got pregnant. Did somebody do something bad to you?"

She sits mute.

"Who made you pregnant?" I insist, moving as close to the scared girl as I dare. "Who?"

Long silence, but she finally lifts her head, looks at me. Her eyes are troubled. No fourteen-year-old eyes should look that way.

"It was my daddy," she whispers.

For a minute I don't speak. I can't speak. The rage exploding inside me is molten. I want that man's neck in my hands. "I just want what's best for my girl," he had said. The same man who violated her, who tortured her life in service to his perversity. I start shaking, trying to control my anger.

"The man in the waiting room who you came with? Is that who you call 'Daddy'? Is he the one who did this to you?"

"Yes," she says. "It's him."

"No one else? No one else has touched you down there? Nobody has done this to you but your daddy? The man you came here with?"

"No one."

"Does your mama know?"

She tightens up, looks down again. One question too many.

"Listen. I won't do an abortion today. We have time to consider that. We won't touch you or deal with your pregnancy. Our first job is to make sure you are safe."

Her head jerks up, fear flaring in her eyes. "He'll hurt me if I don't. I have to! He said if I didn't he'd beat me up again. He will! He's done it before."

"You are a minor," I say. "We have to get you away from him for a while, someplace safe. You are very early in the pregnancy. We can talk again soon, but we have to make you safe."

Her eyes plead with mine. They ask for honesty. They search for an adult to trust.

I reach out, touch her, carefully, very gently. "We'll get you through this. I'm going to have a nurse come sit with you while I make some phone calls. We won't let him hurt you."

Nearly an hour had passed before I felt comfortable leaving the young girl with a nurse and could return to the main office.

"I want to see my girl!" the father demands, as soon as he sees me. His face is red; his hands are clenched in fists.

I keep a lid on my own temper, quell the temptation to scream at him, and instead, impose a cool, professional demeanor.

"It's taking a little longer than we thought," I tell him. "She's young, and we want to be careful. It takes time to prepare such a young patient," I lie. "Try to understand. She's perfectly fine, and we're doing everything to make sure she's safe."

"I want to see her!" he paces back to his seat.

I close the door and hurry to the administrator's office. "We have a reportable incident," I blurt out. "We have to hurry. The girl is a minor, an incest victim. She's identified her father. He's in the waiting room now, but he's really nervous and demanding. He may suspect something. I've told him we've been delayed."

She has the phone in her hand before I finish. We notify both the police and the Child Protection Agency, stress that it's essential for them to synchronize. The girl will be escorted out the back door by a caseworker at the same time the police take the father out the front.

All this takes more time. It's been almost two hours since the girl checked in.

"Where's my girl?" the father demands when I return. "I want to see her!"

I have to physically block him from coming through the door. "Please. Be reasonable," I say. "I'm sorry it's taken so long. We'll be through soon, but it only prolongs things if I have to keep coming out here. It won't be long now."

"I know something is wrong," he accuses. "What's going on?"

He finally storms back to his chair, muttering to himself.

Back with the girl, I fill her in. "People from a place called the Child Protection Agency are coming to pick you up. They are set up to take care of young people who have troubles at home. They'll keep you safe while you figure things out."

"He'll never let them take me," she says.

"The police are coming to ask him some questions. They won't let him hurt you."

The events daze her. By turns she looks relieved, anxious, scared, thankful. The door opens, and the administrator calls me out.

"Everything's set," she says. "The police are coming in."

I get to the waiting room just as they open the door. The father is looking at me, about to speak, when an officer takes his arm.

"What's going on?" he explodes. "What is this?"

"You're coming in for questioning." The officer handcuffs him as they speak.

"My daughter's here. You can't do this."

He shoots me a haunting, burning look. He'll be back, I think. He'll be back, looking for me. I watch just long enough to be convinced they will indeed take him away, then turn and go quickly to the back of the clinic. The girl is just about out the door with the social worker, but I stop them briefly.

"Please come back and talk to me when you feel safe," I say.

She nods distractedly. She looks tiny and vulnerable. A child starting a new life.

I tell the caseworker I'm available any time. I write down my phone numbers. The car drives off.

I have a moment of doubt. I didn't have to probe for the truth. I could have performed the procedure and let her return to her life. It was only through my persistence, and my legal obligation to act on information, that this happened.

In the end, though, it is these cases that make me feel I'm performing the best medicine. It would have been easier not to be thorough, to ignore the red flags. But that extra twenty minutes spent digging for the truth, or explaining something a patient doesn't understand, or answering the hard questions can make a difference for the rest of a woman's life. The moment I simply become a technician performing procedures is the moment I have to quit.

Shortly before the trial of Michael Griffin for the 1993 murder of Dr. David Gunn, former Rev. Paul Hill and 33 others signed what has become known as the "defensive action statement." . . .

We, the undersigned, declare the justice of taking all godly action necessary to defend innocent human life including the use of force. We proclaim that whatever force is legitimate to defend the life of a born child is legitimate to defend the life of an unborn child. We assert that if Michael Griffin did in fact kill David Gunn, his use of lethal force was justifiable provided it was carried out for the purpose of defending the lives of unborn children. Therefore, he ought to be acquitted of the charges against him.

Frederick Clarkson, "Justifiable Homicide: The Signers," Intelligence Report 91 (Summer 1998)

chapter eleven

Irony, if not blatant hypocrisy, is everywhere in the realm of abortion clinics and women's reproductive health. Sexuality is a universal drive, no matter what your ethics are, and a pregnancy is irrefutable. It forces people to confront weaknesses, to face the inconsistencies of their beliefs, conflicts of lifestyle, the disconnect between a public persona and private reality. Or it provokes the powerful temptation to deny and rationalize, to escape that confrontation, whatever it takes.

Sometimes the brazenness of the hypocrisy takes my breath away. In clinics and in protests, we see it every day.

Kathleen was forty-two years old and a model of perfection. Hair, nails, clothes done up as if she were prepped for a high-profile job interview. When I came into the room and asked my standard question, "Are you absolutely sure you want this abortion?" she squared her jaw and glared at me.

"Of course I don't want to have an abortion. I HAVE to have an abortion." She held an oversized purse on her lap, kept fumbling with the latch.

"Why? Is someone forcing you?"

"No one is forcing me. I just CANNOT have a baby now. I know it's murder and should not even be legal, but I HAVE to have an abortion."

"So," I spat back, "if you think this is murder, do you think I am a murderer?"

"Of course you are."

"Do you think I should go to jail for doing abortions?"

"Yes, I do."

I couldn't believe I was hearing this. I felt sick with outrage and disbelief. Maybe I had misunderstood. I asked her again.

"So, you think this should be illegal and that I should go to prison for murder, but you also want me to do an abortion for you?"

"Yes," she said, without blinking an eye.

Everything inside me turned upside down. I had never encountered anything like this.

"I need to step out of the room a minute," I said. I got off my stool and headed for the door.

"You can't leave," she barked. "I want an abortion. It is my right, and you have to do it."

"I have rights, too," I replied, and I slipped through the door. Flashes of the final scene in the movie *If These Walls Could Talk* ran through my head. In the movie, a couple comes to an abortion clinic, supposedly for an abortion. The woman's partner accuses the doctor of being a murderer, then pulls out a gun from a hand bag and kills her. It is a scene burned into my memory.

I paused and took a deep breath before going to talk to the clinic administrator. After I relayed the conversation, I asked that someone else tell the patient that we would not be providing the abortion. There was no way I could do it.

The counselor who had visited with Kathleen earlier went into the room. Within twenty seconds the conflict was loud enough for everyone on the floor to hear.

"I will NOT leave! It is my RIGHT to have an abortion and I am staying until it is DONE!"

Brief silence.

"NO! I will NOT get dressed until I have the ABORTION!"

We heard a loud thump, the patient slamming her fist onto a desk. The clinic administrator called the front desk guard to escort her out. If that didn't work, we'd have to call the police.

"I am going to sue that doctor and this stupid clinic!" the woman yelled. I imagined everyone in the waiting room cringing. I literally hid in the staff lounge until she was gone.

At the end of the day all the staff gathered in the empty recovery room.

"I'm sorry I couldn't confront that woman," I apologized. "It doesn't happen often, but once in a while someone comes along who I simply can't deal with."

We talked about the danger a patient like that could present. From that time on, we established a clinic policy that prevented patients from bringing purses, bulky coats, or bags with them beyond the waiting room.

One of the most galling realities is the lack of consistency within the medical community. In Montana, as in other places, I was repeatedly attacked by anti-choice factions in editorials and letters to the editor. Statements containing false medical information and misleading "facts" went unchecked. Only one physician in Bozeman publicly supported me. The rest either were silent or professed to be against abortion, knuckling under to anti-choice pressure. Yet more than once I was asked to perform a secretive abortion after hours for a girlfriend or wife of a local doctor.

I remember meeting one such doctor at eight PM in the quiet hallway outside my office.

"Thank you for seeing us tonight," he said, shaking my hand. He looked up and down the empty hall. "This is just so awkward, you know."

I kept my thoughts to myself, focused instead on the woman by his side. When I didn't respond, he continued. "Well, at least there's an accountant's office nearby. I can always say we were going there if someone sees us tonight. They work late sometimes, don't they?"

Then there are the patients who come to us, admitting they have been against abortion, but struggling with the uncomfortable fact that they are now the victims of unwanted pregnancies. Suddenly, for them, the black-and-white parameters turn a decided shade of gray.

Early in my career, in a Midwestern clinic, I saw a twenty-two-year-old single mother in the waiting room whom I recognized as one of the group of protesters who had recently chained themselves together with bike locks, blocking the clinic entrance in an attempt to close us down. She had been sitting against the side doors, pounding her fist in a rhythmic way, doing her best to mimic a heartbeat. Thump thud. Thump thud. Thump thud. At the same time she screamed, "Mommy, don't kill me!"

What was she doing in our waiting room? Was she a spy, gathering information? Would she open the doors and let in a flood of protesters? Was she faking a pregnancy in order to find out more about our facilities?

It became clear that she was actually there for an abortion. Unbelievable. The initial reaction from all the staff was anger and disbelief. How dare she expect us to take care of her? Did she take us for fools?

Our most seasoned counselor volunteered to talk with her. The two of them stayed cloistered in the room for perhaps an hour before the counselor reappeared with a look of determination and amazement on her face.

"She really is pregnant and really does want an abortion. I think we should help her, but I also think each of us needs to talk with her first. She should know how we feel about this. More important, she needs to understand the impact she has had on our lives and the lives of our other patients."

There was a lot of resistance from the staff, myself included. The counselor persisted, telling us to be forgiving and understanding and to allow this woman the chance to learn the truth about us and about abortion.

"You never know," she said. "This young woman might end up being an ally. Even if she doesn't, it will be pretty hard for her to go back to the protesters.

"She knows now that things aren't so ethically clear and simple as she was led to believe. Those pat answers aren't working for her. Forget that she was a protester, and listen to her with an open heart."

When I went in to see her, I started with a straightforward question: "Do you believe abortion should be legal?"

"Well, yes, I guess so. Yes. I do. Well, now I do. But I didn't before . . . ," she stumbled over the words.

"What has changed your mind?" I asked.

"This is my second pregnancy. The first time I got pregnant I came here to get an abortion, but the people out front stopped me and promised to help me if I had the baby. They told me I might die in here and that you were awful people that just wanted to kill babies."

I kept listening and prodding her to tell me more.

"They said they'd pay for my prenatal care and give me baby clothes and diapers and all that."

"So you had the baby?" I asked.

"Yes. And I really love him, but he's only five months old, and I am really having a tough time taking care of him. I have to work, but I'd like to go to the community college. I don't know how I could possibly do it with two kids."

"So what happened to the people that promised to help you?"

"All they gave me was a layette set and two boxes of diapers. That's it. They were all friendly and took me to church and wanted me to demonstrate with them, but they really haven't helped me at all with anything. I feel like all they cared about was that I didn't have an abortion."

"But after all the things they told you about us, how do you know who to believe? How could you even dare to come here?" I asked.

"I talked to my aunt. She's a nurse and told me a lot of things I didn't know. I trust her, and she said I should trust you. She said this was a good clinic and that I'd be safe."

I leaned back in my chair, thinking hard about the next thing on my mind. "Tell me," I looked her in the eye. "Are you ever going to protest outside an abortion clinic again?"

"Absolutely not," she replied without hesitation.

"And if your best friend got pregnant and came to you for advice, what would you tell her?" I wasn't going to let up.

"I'd be her friend no matter what. It would be up to her, but I wouldn't try to talk her out of an abortion like I would have last year."

We talked a bit longer. I told her I believed that everything happens for a reason, and that she and I were both learning lessons in forgiveness and understanding.

After the abortion, that young woman became a prochoice advocate. She kept in contact with us. Every time she stopped in, she expressed gratitude for our care and for our ability to see who she really was.

Not all encounters with patients who have been strongly anti-choice end this way. I have had patients who admit that they have been protesters, but rather calmly and rationally explain why they need to end a pregnancy in spite of their beliefs. We give them accurate information and perform safe, legal abortions if they choose to go forward. Some of those same women are back out in front of the clinic protesting within a week of their procedure.

Mostly I'm able to ignore and minimize the impact of protesters, but a few of them make the hair stand up on the back of my neck. Mostly they are men: people who will never experience the personal, agonizing trauma of an unwanted pregnancy but who preach their version of truth, bully patients, and emanate hatred. I'm utterly convinced that, for these people, the abortion issue is not about morality but about power and control. Control over women's lives. Nothing I've observed in them shows any sincere concern or sympathy for children or families.

The first time I saw Chet Gallagher was in Fargo, North Dakota. He was aggressive with patients and staff, swaggering around on the sidewalk in front of the building as if it were his domain. When patients approached, he'd shout in their faces. "You'll die in there," he pointed to the doors. "Your baby will scream in pain. You'll never be able to have another child!"

If a young woman was accompanied by her boyfriend, Gallagher would get in his face, too. "Be a man," he'd yell. "Don't let her do this."

Over the months we learned that Chet Gallagher had been a police officer, a person hired to uphold the law. That he had once been in charge of protecting the public seemed absurd. Here he was breaking laws left and right, racking up many arrests. Over time, he has become one of the national leaders in the anti-choice movement. He now claims to have been arrested more than a hundred times and calls himself a lay minister.

During my years in Bozeman I was targeted by several local men who were obsessed with my clinic. One of them was particularly rabid. He was eventually arrested for trying to burn down the building where my offices were located. Before that, however, he stalked me, put up "wanted" posters with my picture on them, and repeatedly harassed people associated with any aspect of family planning or reproductive health.

At one point he burst into a mother/daughter seminar sponsored by a local medical practice. The weekend session was devoted to fostering family communication and discussing issues of puberty. He rampaged around the room, ranting about teen sex and abortions. He accused the facilitators of fostering promiscuity and loose morals. The facilitators finally had to call the police before the man would leave.

The same man stood up and disrupted church services where some of my employees worshiped, telling the minister and congregation that they were sinners for allowing baby killers in their midst.

The most blatant hypocrisy takes place outside clinics, but inside it isn't uncommon to witness fateful intersections between patients that force them to face their decisions rather than keep them hidden.

One day I heard two very audible gasps in the outer waiting room when a couple of women, both patients with appointments for abortions, came face to face.

"WHAT are YOU doing here?" one of them said.

"I don't know," stammered the other. "What are YOU doing here?"

They stared at each other, both at a loss. The receptionist quickly stepped in and signaled them to follow her to a more private area.

"If the two of you know each other and would like to talk privately, we can provide you with a quiet space. Or one of you can reschedule if you'd like."

They chose to talk. They stayed in there a very long time.

It turned out that they were coworkers at a Catholic school. One of them was an administrator, the other a teacher. No doubt they had each hoped to keep their secret safe and go on with life. The public face they presented to the world could remain unchanged, except for their chance meeting. No doubt they had some rationalizing and explaining to do, but when they came back out, they both seemed resolved and under control.

Both women stayed for their procedures. In fact, they scheduled their follow-up exams for the same day so that they could carpool for the three-hour drive. I have little doubt, given their positions, that they still publicly denounce abortion and tell their students abortion is a grievous sin. Except for their awkward encounter, they might have avoided any confession at all.

For the most part, my knowledge of personal hypocrisy is protected by my commitment to confidentiality. The insights that come to me stay locked up tight by necessity. Occasionally, though, an opportunity comes along to call on someone to live up to public statements.

The first time I turned the tables on the local "crisis pregnancy center," I had a patient in the clinic who really did not want an abortion but who had no resources to cover the costs of prenatal care or childbirth. She was single and without insurance coverage but made just enough money to be ineligible for state assistance. She already had outstanding bills at the hospital and with the local ob-gyn practice. No doctor would see her without payment up front.

We were willing to do the abortion for a reduced rate or for free if necessary. But she really didn't want an abortion. Once I understood her situation, I went to the phone and called the local "crisis pregnancy center."

"Hello, this is Dr. Wicklund."

Dead silence. I might as well have said I was Satan.

"Hello?" I said again. "This is Dr. Wicklund."

"Hello," very tentatively, followed by another long silence.

"I need help with a patient," I said. "She came to me for an abortion, but she really doesn't want one. What she really needs is someone to do her prenatal care and birth for free."

"What do you expect us to do?"

I let that hang for a minute.

"Well, maybe this is your chance to save a baby. Isn't that your mission? Here you are. My suggestion is that you find her the care she needs, or she will be forced to have an abortion."

"But no one does free prenatal care and births."

"How about Dr. Abott? He is always publicly preaching about the evils of abortion. Why don't you call him and see if he'll put his money where his mouth is? Tell him I am willing to do the abortion for free, but it won't be necessary if he can match my offer."

In this case, it worked. Dr. Abott provided her prenatal care and birth without charge, although he reminded her of his noble gesture at every visit. The young woman came by several times to let us know how things were going.

"He always moans about being tricked into the deal," she told us. "Then goes off on these tirades against abortion."

Not surprisingly, the people who pay the greatest price in the abortion war are always the ones without power, without resources, without advocates, the most vulnerable of our culture. Poor women in the United States are four times as likely to have an unwanted pregnancy than affluent women. They are five times more likely to have an unintended birth and three times more likely to have an abortion. The correlation between poverty and unwanted pregnancy is stark.

Too often poor women become pawns in the battle—used while they serve a purpose and abandoned the moment their usefulness ends. People like Martina Greywind.

Fargo, North Dakota. 1992. Martina Greywind is a local figure, one of those people everyone averts their eyes from on the street. Her hands are weathered, her hair disheveled. Her face is creased with the lines of her life's trials—winters spent sleeping on heat grates and mattresses of newspaper, repeated physical abuse, excessive alcohol and drug use. You'd guess she was fifty, but she is twenty-eight years old.

She regularly sniffs paint. Her face is often flecked with gold from spray paint cans. She is no stranger to jail.

She is pregnant and wants an abortion. She has already given birth to six children, cares for none of them. For weeks she has been manically sniffing paint, not simply to get high but in hopes that she will provoke a miscarriage.

Now she is in jail again, charged with recklessly endangering her fetus, sentenced to an ironic nine-month term. She makes no secret of her desire to obtain an abortion.

In her cellblock two members of the Lambs of Christ are also incarcerated, held for their illegal actions against the local clinic. They hound her with rhetoric. "Don't kill your baby," they shout. "We will help you. Your baby will be loved."

Martina tells them to leave her alone, that it is none of their business, but they persist. For weeks I am kept abreast of the case through clinic staff. I make it clear that I'm willing to come to Fargo if Martina is able to have an abortion.

The story makes local daily headlines: "Greywind Still Wants Abortion." The *New York Times* picks up the story. Her plight is featured on the *Today Show*.

When a local resident offers to cover Greywind's abortion costs, the Lambs of Christ accuse the clinic of bribery. They raise $11,000 and offer it to Greywind if she will continue her pregnancy. She rejects them.

Then Martina is sentenced to thirty days of rehabilitation in a state hospital more than a hundred miles away. Authorities refuse to transport her for medical appointments, saying it is a waste of taxpayer money. By the time she returns, it will be too late for an abortion. A last-minute court order delays her rehabilitation sentence for a few days.

Martina requests a leave for a clinic appointment. It is granted for Sunday. The clinic is normally closed on weekends, but the staff agrees to be available. I will fly in from Milwaukee. When the antis get wind of this, they go wild. Desecrating the Sabbath, they cry. We will stop this!

They go to court for an injunction, claiming Greywind is mentally incompetent. They are rejected.

I follow the drama from afar. It becomes clear to me that there is no way we will succeed on the publicly announced day. Too much fervor has built up. The antis will stop at nothing.

"We have to change the day," I tell the administrator by phone.

"But it's already Thursday," she says. "We have to go to court to do that. There isn't time."

"We need to try," I persist. "Otherwise it'll be a circus, a standoff, and Martina will be trapped in the middle."

The clinic administrator goes to the city attorney. "Lives are at stake here," she tells him. "If we go ahead on Sunday, there is no telling what might happen."

He agrees to try, but the presiding judge is away on vacation. Finally we reach the judge by phone and get his verbal agreement. The court order is filed seconds before the office closes on Friday. We can only hope that the antis haven't gotten wind of the change.

On Friday night, after a full day of clinic in Milwaukee, I fly to Fargo. Before boarding the plane I call Sonja.

"Hi Sonja. How was school today?" We talk about the day. I try to sound reassuring, but Sonja knows something is up. "Listen, I won't be able to get home tonight. I have to fly to Fargo for a special case. I'll be home by tomorrow afternoon, okay?" I can hear the disappointment in her voice, but she bucks up as she always does. "I'm sorry, sweetie. It's important, or I wouldn't go. Tell Randy what's going on. I love you."

It is nearly midnight when I slip in the back door of a Fargo hotel and register under a false name. My sleep is restless, but at six-thirty AM I meet a van at the back door. The clinic director and lab tech are already in the vehicle.

At the same time, two volunteers drive to the garage at the Fargo jail. Martina climbs behind the back seat and hides under blankets. They make their way to the clinic.

The Lambs of Christ still in jail somehow get the word and raise the alarm, but they are too late. Martina is already inside the clinic offices by the time protesters start swarming around outside like angry insects. Police cars pull up. The media arrives, sniffing the next headline.

Inside, Martina and I sit in a small room. I turn a radio on to help drown out the shouts and commotion from the street.

"How are you holding up?" I ask her.

"I'm tired. I just want this to be over," she replies quietly.

She reminds me of a rag doll. Pliable. Soft. Plain. No grit or fight left in her. I want to take her home and try to make everything better for her, but I know I am not being realistic. We move forward.

"Are you absolutely sure this is what you want to do?" I ask.

She just nods, but her head is down, and she is not looking at me. I wait for more. She nods again. Still I say nothing. Finally, she raises her head and looks at me.

"Yes," she says in a very soft voice.

The staff wants me to hurry. They are justifiably afraid of the growing crowd and mounting tension outside.

But Martina and I move at our own pace. We are together in a different realm, oddly serene. The procedure goes well, but instead of moving her to the recovery room right away, I just roll my stool up beside her and place my hand on her arm. We are both silent. We each shed tears we don't acknowledge. I feel the weight of her life, the fatigue in her bones. I stand; our eyes meet.

The news appeal swirling around Martina dries up and disappears in no time. Within days the charges against her are dropped, and she is released.

Her "protectors" no longer find her useful. They claim they were tricked and misled by the clinic, as if they ever had a right to be part of Martina Greywind's decision. Never once, before or after her abortion, do they make any genuine attempt to change the circumstances of her life. She slips back to the streets, becomes anonymous again, a cultural pariah.

The ultimate and most threatening expression of hypocrisy comes from the segment of the "pro-life" movement that believes murdering abortion doctors is "justifiable homicide." The biblical commandment "Thou shalt not kill" is conveniently glossed over in their ends-justify-the-means philosophy. They spout religion, they pay homage to godliness, they call themselves god-fearing, yet they find it in their hearts to commit murder, arson, and violence of every kind against doctors and clinics.

I remember the first time I saw Sonja shrink away in horror from someone who innocently announced their devotion to Christianity. To her, Christians were the people who called me a killer and who publicly agitated for the murder of her mother.

Until the courts ordered them to cease, the justifiable homicide crowd maintained a website listing every known abortion provider in the country, along with addresses, phone numbers, information about other family members, photos, and personal profiles. It was called the Nuremberg File, and it was nothing less than a detailed hit list. If a doctor was wounded or killed, that entry would be highlighted in a different color on the site, as if to check off a job well done.

Seeing myself and my family listed on that website threw a dark shadow across my basic assumption of human goodness.

FOR SALE:
Women's Reproductive Health Care solo practice. Have been providing first trimester abortions and general women's health care including family planning and annual exams. Located in Bozeman, Montana: college town of 30,000 surrounded by mountains and clean air. Call Mountain Country Women's Clinic for details.

In 2006, 87 percent of counties in the United States had no abortion provider.

chapter twelve

I was finding it hard to breathe. I flipped through the pages of the patient chart. The symptoms were all there, plain as day—hormone levels off, weak spells, headaches. Evidence stretching back more than eight years. Why hadn't these been investigated? Why hadn't I caught them? This patient had suffered because of my inattention, my failure.

Worse yet, I had made a conscious decision to remain at a distance in this case. I had vowed to be a daughter, not a doctor.

Dad sat on the exam table, swinging his legs. I had scheduled this visit from Montana to coincide with the follow-up appointment after the surgery to remove his brain tumor, a tumor that could have been identified and removed years earlier. The doctor hadn't come in yet. I had power of attorney over Dad's medical affairs, so I was justified in looking at his charts.

The doctor in me was horrified at the implications of this inattention. The daughter in me kept staring at the symptoms and complaints, shaking my head, thinking of all he had suffered through and missed out on over those years.

It had come to a head five months earlier. I had been visiting Sonja at her college in Boston when I got an urgent message to call home. "Family emergency" was all I knew when I dialed the number for my sister, Julie.

"Julie," I said, when she answered.

"Sue. Dad's in the hospital," her voice was all business. "He had another severe headache, but this time he was completely confused and acting really strange. He was very weak, like those spells he gets out of the blue. His labs are all out of whack. Sue, they say he might die. Soon."

I felt myself shift into medical crisis-management mode. "What tests have they done?" I asked.

"Well," Julie said, "besides the blood tests, they took an MRI of his head, but it's Friday afternoon, and there won't be a radiologist in until Monday."

"You're telling me that Dad's dying and no one can evaluate an MRI for days?"

"Yes. That's exactly what I'm telling you."

"I'm catching the next plane. Get your hands on those films and meet me at the airport. I know someone in radiology at Abbott Hospital. We'll get them read right away."

Several hours later, driving through Minneapolis traffic, I thought about a doctor visit two years earlier. Dad's headaches and weak spells had already been going on for more than five years. He had been losing weight, acting inappropriately, experiencing memory loss. By then he was taking an alarming number of medications. I had begged the doctor to do an MRI of Dad's head but was told it was unnecessary. I just needed to accept the fact that Dad was aging and that these symptoms were nothing more than a normal decline in an elderly man. My intuition told me otherwise, but I had acquiesced, stayed out of meddling in his medical affairs, held myself rigidly to my daughter role.

Mom had urged me to get more involved. I wished now that I had listened to her. Now we finally had an MRI to study, but it might be too late. Dad was incoherent, incontinent, close to death in the intensive care unit of a tiny rural hospital.

"This is a pituitary tumor," the radiologist said, pointing to a dark, spherical anomaly on the films, just behind the optic nerve. "Pretty obvious. And it fits the medical history you've given me. Given its size and the duration of his symptoms, I'd say this tumor has been here a while."

Even to the untrained eye, the tumor was obvious, glaring. For me, it was an accusation.

When the pituitary gland is shut down or destroyed, the rest of the endocrine system malfunctions as well. Without hormones, you die. In Dad's case we were lucky. Within a month his condition stabilized, and he was able to have brain surgery to have the tumor removed.

"Looking at the size of that schnoz," the surgeon had joked, "I'd say this procedure will be a breeze. We'll just drive right in through that nasal cavity and pluck out the tumor."

In fact, the surgery was a difficult but successful one. Dad's face looked like it had been flattened by a truck, but he healed quickly.

It was February now. I'd come back to Wisconsin to take Dad personally to his follow-up exam. No more distancing myself from his medical care. From now on, I'd be paying strict attention to the details. I would become a regular presence in my parents' lives. I also hoped to take part in the annual family tradition of tapping trees and making maple syrup.

Lurking in the background was the state of Mom's health. Dad was rebounding nicely, putting weight back on. He called himself "the new, old man." He could once again do chores, walk in the woods, play cribbage, participate in conversations. His familiar sense of humor reemerged. The most heart-wrenching part of his recovery was filling him in on the events he'd missed, things that happened over recent years that he didn't remember, including the death of his son-in-law.

Mom, on the other hand, had been weak and tired for several months. We took her to the Mayo Clinic, where she was diagnosed with Myelodysplastic Syndrome with sideroblastic anemia. In English, it meant that her bone marrow didn't properly mature her red blood cells, among other things. Average life expectancy following this diagnosis is two years.

I'd blown it with Dad. He and my family had paid a heavy price. I wasn't about to let the same thing happen with Mom. Still, I knew exactly what that meant. In order to truly care for Mom and be there on the medical scene, I'd have to consider moving back to the Midwest.

Like the patients who came every day to my Montana clinic, I confronted my life choice: whether to pursue my career and ambition or put that on hold, perhaps forever; how to be my own person and also be a responsible family member; how to come to a decision I could live with.

I was still coming to grips with the failure of my second marriage. There was no terrible disagreement or ulterior motive for the divorce. Randy is a good, kind man. We've remained friends, and he continues to be Randad to Sonja, keeping in contact and seeing her frequently. A large part of our decision to part ways was based on our inability to reconcile our geographic separation. We had each developed our own lives. Randy was well along in his engineering career, and I had my place in the West. Once Sonja graduated from high school and went off to college, we made the divorce official.

I had told Randy that I would never come back to Wisconsin. "Never" was a word I often told my patients to be very careful with. Many times women have told me that they would never have believed they would find themselves in an abortion clinic. Now I was faced with my own careless use of that inflexible word.

And, like for many of my abortion patients, none of it felt black-and-white. Where they weighed the responsibilities and rewards of being a parent against life's realities, I struggled with the closure at the other end of life, and the duty I had to help ease that transition and make what time remained as full and vital as possible for people I loved.

For the next ten months I tried to do both. I had worked so hard to create a clinic that reflected my beliefs and convictions, to serve women the way they deserved to be served. My staff had developed into a competent, supportive, effective team. I felt somewhat responsible for their futures. Our service to women who came from as far away as Canada and the Dakotas addressed an urgent need. We had developed a reputation based on compassion and respect. I couldn't bear to give that up.

From February to December I flew back and forth from Montana to Wisconsin, spending several days a week operating the clinic, then returning to my family. Life was a whirlwind of competing demands. As the weeks passed, more and more things slipped through the cracks. Try as I might, I couldn't maintain the juggling act.

On New Year's Eve 1997, I was sitting alone in the hot tub on Julie's porch in Wisconsin. Steam swirled around me. Winter woods surrounded the house. I couldn't stop crying. My tears were a confused blend of self-pity, sadness for my parents, and guilt and anger over giving up my clinic. I was terrified of losing my autonomy, my sense of self. Above all, I knew that I had to come home and stay home, and that it meant ending my work at the clinic in Montana.

I had been putting out feelers for someone who might buy the clinic and keep the practice open. I had some nibbles, and two serious inquiries, but the business didn't generate enough money to finalize a deal. In the end, I had to close down Mountain Country Women's Clinic, five years to the day from the proud morning it opened. In February 1998 I closed that door for the last time.

At that moment an overwhelming sadness engulfed me. On some level it felt like a betrayal of Dr. Balice's commitment to keeping the clinic open, and a betrayal of my staff. It felt as if I were turning my back on a part of myself.

Before I left for Wisconsin, I bought a small, primitive cabin on some acreage about forty miles east of Bozeman. No running water. The only electricity came through an extension cord from the power post. Plenty of sagebrush and mountain-filled skyline. It was a quiet, windswept, austere, beautiful, lonely spot. More important, it was my deposit on a future out west, something tangible and real in a life now so full of unknowns.

•

In a way, caring for Mom and Dad took me back to my time as a single parent caring for a toddler. Days melted away in a blur of tending to details, treading water, doing repetitive chores. Trips to the pharmacy, doctor appointments, keeping the house clean, doing laundry, making phone calls, keeping track of medications, and always watching for changes in Mom's condition. It was exhausting and consuming, as well as important and satisfying, but I often felt that I'd done nothing of significance for weeks at a stretch. Julie and I became a parent-care team, and we developed a sense for when the other person was overloaded.

I had to tamp down the ache I felt for Montana, for my clinic and my work. The Midwestern humidity gnawed at my joints, slowed me down. I kept glancing to the horizon, willing mountains to be there. But I couldn't let myself dwell on it. I'd made my commitment.

Although Dad had substantially recovered physically, his mental lapses didn't disappear. Mom's health was truly precarious, but we couldn't afford not to keep an eye on Dad. We would send him to town with a grocery list, and he'd return an hour later with stories of the people he'd seen, but no food. When he was home alone with Mom, he would sometimes get so preoccupied with a chore in the barn that he'd completely forget she might need his help.

Mom had weekly lab tests at the clinic. Within a year she needed frequent blood transfusions. Her disease weakened her bones to the point that she started having spontaneous fractures of her spine, then her hip and one leg. She became wheelchair-bound, had to be helped to the toilet and into bed. We moved her into the old dining room during the day so she could be close to the hub of the kitchen. The old living room became their bedroom. The upstairs rooms went vacant. Her pain became almost impossible to control. And she was angry.

Once we were at the hospital getting a blood transfusion when one of her old schoolmates happened to walk by. He stopped and came in the room.

"Vera," he said. "So good to see you. How are you doing?"

She never looked up at him, kept her head bowed. "Oh, I'm alright," she mumbled.

"It must be hard to see people your age who are healthy," I said, after he left.

"I'm so angry that this happened!" she blurted out. "My friends are out playing golf, spending time with their families, going places. Look at me. It's not fair!" She hunched over, her muscles tight, her hands clenched into fists.

I did look at her. The sight made me grieve. This is what had replaced the retirement my parents had looked forward to, this purgatory full of pain and dependence.

Days marched past, weeks, years. Mom's condition steadily worsened, but Julie and I were very attentive. Every change was monitored, medications adjusted, quirks checked out. She outlived her prognosis. We hired a compassionate, cheerful local woman to help out several days a week. Dad was cantankerous with her and resented having a stranger in the house. Fact was, we desperately needed the help. The smallest chores had become ordeals.

Flower Grandma was still alive, suffering from Alzheimer's disease, living in her third nursing home. She and I had never again discussed her childhood friend. I don't know if, in her later years, she even remembered the trauma. We tried to explain Mom's situation to her. She seemed to understand. It had been months since they'd seen each other.

On a sunny spring day I picked up Flower Grandma and drove her to my parents' home. The farms were green with new crops. Flocks of Canada geese flew over the fields.

"Oh!" she exclaimed. "Big birds."

When we passed farm silos, she'd count them off. "One, two, three silos," she said. "One, two, three, four, five silos." Her obsessive behavior was symptomatic of Alzheimer's. On one level her habit was cute and endearing. On another, a chilling sign of a mind trying desperately to hang on to some thread of control.

At the house I helped Flower Grandma from the car. She shuffled her way in through the doorway she had entered hundreds of times over the decades. Some spark of recognition lit her face. We moved farther into the house, to the old dining room. Mom lay there on her hospital bed. In that moment I saw her truly for what she'd become, a shrunken, diminished husk of herself.

"NO!" Flower Grandma shouted at the sight of her daughter. "Not . . . not . . . oh no!"

I pulled her into the kitchen and made coffee—my ingrained response to stress. We sat together at the table in silence, cradling the warm mugs. Crying. Eventually she was able to walk back into the room, holding her coffee cup, and sit with Mom.

On the trip back to the nursing home, Flower Grandma counted silos, looking out across the land so familiar and yet so foreign. She died that spring, just after Easter. Bucking tradition, her six granddaughters were her pallbearers.

I went back to work part-time for a clinic owned by a large corporation in St. Paul. The two-hour commute became my island of calm and solitude. I could listen to books on tape, play music, let my thoughts wander uninterrupted, simply be alone without demands or distractions. I loved being with patients again and got completely pulled in by their circumstances.

At this job, however, I was no longer the boss, and I had little opportunity to have an impact on policies or protocols. Decisions about patient care, staffing, and individual concerns were dictated by a hierarchy that I often couldn't understand and that seemed unapproachable. I was continually getting into trouble for rocking the boat, for questioning the wisdom of rules, and for putting patient requests above rigid guidelines.

•

"Hi, I'm Dr. Wicklund. How are you doing, Kelly?"

"Why can't my mom be here with me?" she asked.

She was sixteen but looked twelve. She clutched a stuffed animal and slumped in her chair. Her eyes were pleading, young, afraid. What she needed, more than any other thing, was the comfort that her mother, and only her mother, could provide.

I clenched up. It was so clear that a mother should be allowed to join her daughter through this process if that was what they both wanted. Yet it was counter to clinic policy. I had gone through appropriate channels and requested that, in some cases, rules be bent in response to unique circumstances. I had been consistently rebuffed. Only staff could be with a patient during an abortion: end of discussion.

Kelly's mom and the seventeen-year-old boyfriend sat off by themselves in the waiting room. When I went to visit with them, the mother immediately put her hand on my arm and begged to be with Kelly. Her eyes were mirrors of her daughter's.

"Please, Dr. Wicklund, let me come in with her. She is so young. So scared. I can help her through this."

"It's against regulations," I sighed. "But listen, I'm a mother, too. I understand your desire." What I was really thinking of was my parents and my compelling need to be included in the decisions and procedures that affected their lives. More than that, the need to be watching them, holding their hands, reading their body language—that language only someone close would understand.

"Listen," I said, with sudden resolve. "In just a minute I'll get up and walk into the surgical area. I want you to get up and follow me. Look like you know exactly what you're doing and where you're going. Just follow me."

I waited until I saw the clinic manager go into her office and close the door; then I stood and walked through the waiting room into the surgical area. Kelly's mom was right on my heels when we entered the room where my assistant was waiting. She immediately went to her daughter and hugged her.

"Your mom can be with you," I told Kelly, "but please don't mention this to any of the patients you see in the re-covery room. When the abortion is over, your mom will stay in this room until we can slip her back to the waiting area."

The procedure went smoothly. Kelly needed lots of TLC. Her mother was a tremendous help. She pressed her face against her daughter's, quietly sang her a song, kissed her tear-streaked face.

At my clinic, as in many of the smaller, independent clin-ics I'd worked in, we made decisions like this on an individ-ual basis. In some cases it is extremely helpful to have a partner or husband or parent with the patient. Many times it would not be the best thing. In St. Paul, we were discour-aged from assessing cases on an individual basis and repri-manded for bending the rules.

At the end of the day I was called to the manager's office. My infraction had come to her attention. She wasn't interested in the extenuating circumstances, the fact that a patient's experience had been eased by having her mother with her. That wasn't the point. The point was that I had disobeyed policy.

I felt like a school kid in the principal's office. I took my reprimand, but I didn't apologize. Nor did I promise never to bend the rules. My priorities were clear. I kept remembering my own mother's tears when she learned about my abortion and wanted so badly to be with me. My experience would have been so different had she been there. There are times when corporate guidelines and efficiency are secondary to the needs of a family going through transition. For me, ignoring individual circumstances was unacceptable.

•

Resuming work at a clinic was a relief, but my true refuge was in Montana. Whenever I could carve out some time to take a break, I would drive nonstop to my cabin retreat. Each time I had to overcome the burden of guilt for leaving Julie behind to take the load.

Once there, I might stay in pajamas for days. Hours at a time I sat on the deck and stared out at the mountains, holding an unopened novel on my lap. Time flowed past me. Dry winds stroked my face. The open space made me breathe deep, drink in the view, wallow in the long silences.

I began to meet my neighbors on the ranches and in houses scattered across the landscape. Some of them would become my best friends. They got to know me, listened to my stories, shared their own. Every time I came back, I settled in more comfortably and quickly. More and more, it was becoming home.

Sadly, we weren't able to care for Mom at home to the end. She needed blood transfusions every two weeks. Transportation to the hospital had become intolerable. Putting her in an extended care facility adjacent to the hospital was our only recourse. The small hospital was very supportive of our family efforts. We were included in medical discussions and decisions. Staff welcomed our help.

Much of the time we simply sat at her bedside, waiting for whatever might come up, just being in her company. Toward the end, she lapsed into long periods of semi-consciousness, more than sleep. As I sat through the hours, I started drawing plans for remodeling my Montana cabin.

Mom never reconciled herself to her fate. Her bitterness, so uncharacteristic, made me ache for her. We were always on call. More than once I had to turn around on a Montana-bound trip to tend to the latest crisis. She had been terminally ill for more than five years. I had put my life on hold for half a decade already. And Dad's Alzheimer's symptoms were becoming undeniable.

He would forget where he was, why he'd come someplace, who he was talking to. At least he could still play a cunning game of cribbage, but we learned not to challenge him when he bent the rules here and there. He developed an alarming habit of taking off in his car and driving aimlessly around on the rural roads. We'd get calls from people who'd seen Dad's car twenty miles away. As Mom's life wound down, we started Dad on a new regimen of medications specifically targeting his Alzheimer's symptoms.

January 2003. Mom had been in a light coma for three days. She hadn't eaten but had roused enough to sip some liquids. These spells had been going on for the last month. Her lucid periods were rare and fleeting. Most of the time she was incoherent, confused, weak. Her pain was so intense that she required large doses of morphine. Her bones were so fractured we could no longer turn her. Her kidneys were shutting down.

On a Monday morning, her lab day, I got a call from the doctor.

"The only reason we would do labs is to see if she is low enough on hemoglobin to qualify for Medicaid to pay for a transfusion on Wednesday," he said.

"If we don't give her blood, she'll die," I whispered.

"Sue, your mom is dying right now."

In the end, we decided to forgo the labs and provide comfort measures only. Let her go. The words kept running in the background. It's time. Let her go.

Then, on Tuesday morning, Mom opened her eyes, looked around, wanted something to eat. She asked what day it was.

"It's Tuesday, Mom." I knew what the next question would be, and I dreaded it.

"Am I getting my three units of blood on Wednesday?"

"Mom," I said, "you've been completely out of it for four days. We didn't do your labs."

Silence. She knew exactly what I was saying.

"Are you just letting me die?" she accused. "I want the labs, and I want the blood, and that's that."

I called the doctor, who came right over. Despite his explanation she insisted on the transfusion. Mom demanded to sit up in a wheelchair. She hadn't been out of bed in weeks. She placed herself with her back to me while she spoke to the doctor. I felt like an abject failure.

We did as she asked, but her lucidity lasted only a few hours. She lapsed again into a restless coma.

Sonja was with her when she died, early one January morning. Most of the family had gathered around her the night before, telling stories, being together. Some of us hadn't seen each other in years. Mom lay motionless, but her vital signs reacted to the sounds of our voices. I knew that on some level she was aware of us, responding to us.

At dawn, just before death, she roused, became very restless. Everyone but Sonja and one of her cousins had gone home. Mom was trying to say something. Sonja leaned close. She wanted desperately to make it out. Mom was very frustrated, repeatedly struggled to form words. She died with Sonja still bent over her, still trying to hear.

Four days later I was with Dad at the house, getting him ready for the funeral.

"Dad, you have to get dressed up and look nice."

"For what?" he demanded.

"Dad, it's Mom's funeral."

"Oh my gosh," he turned to me. "Vera? When did she die?"

We drove in silence to the service, through the winter, rural countryside. Crows flew over the brown stubble in farm fields. At one point I looked over and caught Dad whispering to himself, counting out a row of silos as we passed.

Between 1982 and 2000, the number of abortion providers in the United States declined from 2,900 to 1,819, a drop of 37 percent, and the trend has continued since. In 2004, almost 60 percent of abortion providers were more than fifty years old.

— chapter thirteen

After Mom died, it took months for my head to clear. For the better part of a decade she had been my focus, my job, my preoccupation. Now she was gone, but I was reminded of her everywhere. Almost daily I caught myself thinking of a task I needed to do for her. Or I'd pick up the phone to call her about something on my mind. Then, like waking from a dream, I snapped back to reality, a life without her in it. Sonja had lived in Ecuador during the last year, and I'd felt some of the same sense of disorientation and loss, but I could call Sonja, send her a letter, imagine her living an adventure.

Mom was simply gone. All that remained was her memory, the material things that were part of her life, the family and friends she touched. Alternately, I was angry, relieved, confused, terribly sad.

I kept working in St. Paul, providing state-mandated informed consent counseling and abortions. It was my sanctuary, my escape. As always, I became completely absorbed in patients' situations. My involvement was immediate, physical, all consuming. One at a time I engaged with them while I let the rest of the world spin in its orbit without me. The only interruptions came when some administrative snag or financial policy would divert our interaction or stop us cold.

The work was my haven, as it always has been, but the fact was, I was worn down, adrift, unable to see my way clear to a future.

Over Mother's Day, four months after Mom died, I took a backpack trip to Arizona. I hiked alone into the dry mountains outside of Tucson. For days I pushed myself physically, wandering the austere high country while the pulses of grief and loss worked through me. There in the desert air, I started writing a letter to Mom. I let all the anger and lost years and love and mourning flow onto the scribbled pages, one after another.

Even after the trip was over, I kept reworking the letter, editing it, adding to it. Weeks later, when it was done, when I felt drained of those emotions, I burned it, one page at a time. In the rising curls of smoke I truly began the process of letting her go.

All that summer I traveled back and forth between Montana and Wisconsin. I continued to provide abortions at least six days out of every month, but my focus was on building a house out of the cabin on my property, the place I'd been drawing by Mom's bedside. I learned to use carpentry tools—plumb bobs, levels, table saws, nail guns. I peeled logs, helped raise walls, stacked and carried endless piles of lumber.

I lived in my van, parked on a rise with panoramic views of the mountains and sky. I slept with the doors open, woke in the darkness to the star-pricked sky and the howls of coyotes. The smell of sage filled my head. I took showers at the neighbors', sat for hours by the small stream across the field, cooked meals on a camp stove with the healing scenery for my dining room. I was coming back to life.

But then I'd return to Wisconsin, to the guilt and weight of responsibility there. Dad was steadily losing his grip negotiating life. He was becoming a challenge for Julie. At one point I decided to bring Dad back to Montana with me for two weeks, more to give Julie a break than to give Dad a vacation. He couldn't get comfortable. He lost his bearings, never understood why he was sleeping in a neighbor's trailer I'd pulled over to my property. Several days into his stay he announced that he was heading home, even if he had to walk all the way.

In Wisconsin he was still living on his own in the family house, but he needed daily supervision and care. He was angry much of the time, disoriented and feeble. We got him a dog, thinking he'd welcome the company, but he'd forget to feed it, get confused about whose pet it was. We finally had to take it away.

Much to the horror of some of my relatives, it was time to reckon with Dad's collection of guns. They had been the passion of so much of his life, but they were simply too dangerous for him to be around. There were eight loaded guns in the bedroom alone, more in the kitchen, one in the bathroom. We cleaned out every gun we could find, hundreds of them, the collection of a lifetime, the legacy of the vibrant, funny, skilled, strong man who had been my father.

Would I have to spend another decade stuck in neutral?

As fall approached, I wrapped up the building project as best I could and moved back to the Midwest for the winter. Dad's needs were a daily challenge, much as Mom's had been. Julie and I cooked his meals, did his laundry, cleaned house, kept up his medications, took him to doctor appointments. I felt myself slide back into that caregiving mode, with all its conflicts and frustrations.

On top of that, things began to change at work.

I was being scheduled for fewer and fewer days. I suspected that it was the consequence of my outspokenness on patient care issues and bureaucratic protocols. In some cases I had appealed to my superiors. When that went nowhere, I several times contacted higher authorities. In every instance, they eventually agreed with me and overruled the lower management. My determination to be a vocal patient advocate was rubbing someone wrong. While the clinic staff were completely supportive and competent, they didn't have any more power than I did.

About that time, several insurance companies started to deny payment for abortions that weren't performed by a doctor with a board-certified specialty. Reproductive health is not a specialty with board certification. Suddenly I was the doctor on staff with more experience and a lower rate of complications than most, but limited by managed care rules. The accumulating stress at work began to erode the satisfaction I found with patients.

For another year I yo-yoed back and forth from Montana to Wisconsin, from one life I craved to another I felt obligated to. I knew I had to make a living, but I also knew I couldn't keep up my fractured existence and endure the emotional tug of war. By that time we'd hired people to help take care of Dad, who was still living in his home.

I loved seeing my western home come together. I spent hours planting flower beds and trees. While I gardened, I started toying with the possibility of pursuing other work.

I spent time with a career counselor who identified what she perceived were my strengths, and encouraged me to consider new directions.

Along with a friend, I experimented with using my home and property as a retreat center for caregivers and social activists. We held several retreats, but it was very expensive and I couldn't face the fund-raising challenge it would take to pull it off. I talked to a local veterinarian I respected about being his assistant. I looked for jobs in the medical field on the Internet, but I couldn't get excited about a career devoted to managing high blood pressure. For a time I entered a partnership with some neighbors who ran a pottery business, making and marketing pottery funeral urns.

All the while the prospect of abandoning my profession, and the society of abortion providers, nagged at me.

One evening I spontaneously called up a colleague, the woman who had been chief resident at the hospital where I did my internship. She had been my first teacher in the practice of providing abortions. I admitted to her that I was considering other lines of work. She wasn't surprised. She didn't condemn me. She knew only too well how profound and personal the issues were. Perhaps I was looking for some kind of confirmation, maybe even permission, to move on, try something new, call it good. I didn't get that either.

Instead, our conversation drifted to the other providers we knew, how they coped with the stress and danger, and to a discussion about the violence we face and the emotional price we pay.

I told her that I had been thinking lately about a memorial service in Pensacola, Florida, back in March 1994, marking the first anniversary of Dr. Gunn's murder. Abortion doctors came to the service from all over North America, along with clinic directors, political activists, members of his family. Many of us wore bulletproof vests. A man named Paul Hill hung around the fringes. We knew him as an anti-abortion activist. I was very spooked by him, but most people thought he was harmless; some even engaged him in small talk.

As it turned out, Paul Hill murdered an abortion doctor just months after Dr. Gunn's memorial. On July 29, 1994, Hill shot Dr. John Britton at a clinic in Florida. Hill came to the clinic before Britton's police escort arrived. He first killed Britton's bodyguard, retired Air Force Lt. Colonel James Barrett, with a shotgun, then shot Dr. Britton in the head.

My former chief resident and I talked about the strain of working in isolation. An occasional conference or regional meeting will pull colleagues briefly together, but for the most part, we live our lives, figure out how to survive, serve our patients, and fashion the strategies that allow us to keep going alone.

After the phone call I continued to dwell on Dr. Gunn's memorial. It had been very clear that each doctor had coping mechanisms, had structured living situations and relationships to accommodate this profession, and had individual motivations that kept him or her working. No matter the differences in style, the lines each of us wouldn't cross, and the reasons behind our choices, there was also an unequivocal sense of mutual respect and solidarity present in that gathering.

Early in my career, I had occasionally called my mentor, Jane Hodgson, the doctor who had taught me so much. Dr. Hodgson died in 2006 at the age of ninety-one. She was a legend in the field of women's reproductive health and lived on the raw edge of the battle. She was also a gentle and soft-spoken woman, with clear insights and quiet authority. Whenever I had a unique case—a difficult fibroid or cyst, a woman with a systemic illness that might complicate things, a patient with an unusually tight cervix—I'd call to discuss my approach.

Inevitably, those phone conversations went beyond simple procedural advice. In the margins, we also talked through my motivations, the realities of the path I'd chosen, the impacts on my personal and emotional life. Over time, though, as I became more experienced, those calls diminished, then ceased.

Later, before she died too young of a brain tumor, I used to call Dr. Liz Karlin. I had helped train her so she could take over for me at the clinic in Appleton, Wisconsin, and she was an outspoken advocate for women's rights. She lessened the gravity of my situation with her irreverence and humor. She was once quoted in an op-ed story as saying, "Until abortion rights in this country are assured, no penis should be allowed to enter another woman!"

The solace of phone contacts and an occasional meeting can't overcome the reality that I am part of a far-flung culture within the medical community. We are outcasts, bonded by our commitment, valued and shunned for our services. Each of us manages our personal high-wire act. It is a solitary show. From time to time we hear about each other. Almost always, when we do, it's bad news.

Dr. Tiller, for example, who runs a clinic in Wichita, Kansas. He endures the daily barrage of picketers, puts up with the mundane, but onerous, harassment. He and other doctors who work at his clinic are followed home by picketers. Their families are hassled, their neighborhoods leafleted.

One day in 1993, Dr. Tiller was in his car in the parking lot outside his clinic when he noticed a woman approaching. He recognized her as one of the Lambs of Christ. She strode up to his car window, pulled out a gun, and shot him. Dr. Tiller only had time to raise his arms over his head. The bullet went through both arms, but missed his skull.

The very next day, Dr. Tiller returned to his clinic and went back to work.

"I was really lucky," he told me. "It was a small-caliber gun, and she was a lousy shot."

Dr. Leroy Carhartt, from Nebraska, began providing abortions after retiring from surgical practice and a twenty-one-year career in the Air Force. As a young doctor, while abortions were still illegal, he had seen hundreds of women in surgical wards, many in critical condition, some dying, from botched and illegal abortions. At the end of his working life, instead of retiring, he took up clinic work out of his belief that women should be able to have safe and professional abortions.

In the fall of 1991, his home and horse barn were set on fire and completely gutted. Carhartt escaped in his car with only the clothes he was wearing. Seventeen horses, and several family pets, perished in the flames. Despite the fact that the fire was started simultaneously from seven different locations on his property, no arson charges were ever filed. The next day, Dr. Carhartt received a letter from an abortion protester who compared the death of his horses to the "murder" of babies in clinics.

In response, Dr. Carhartt increased his practice from part-time to full-time. Even now he refuses to wear a bullet-proof vest. "The antis know enough by now to just shoot for the head," he says.

Not every doctor, and not every family, can take the strain. A physician I knew in southern Wisconsin quit providing abortions in response to the anti-choice tactics directed at his family. The protesters followed his wife to the hairdresser, where they harangued her and the other clients.

They picketed the garage where he had his car serviced, followed his kids to school, hung posters around town accusing him of murder. In the end, it was too much. His family couldn't stand the pressure. Who could blame them? He made a public announcement that he would stop providing abortions.

Dr. Warren Hern operates a clinic in Boulder, Colorado. His clinic has been one of those targeted by Operation Rescue. Randall Terry, the national leader of that organization, publicly prayed for Hern's death during the protest. One day five bullets were fired through the front office window.

He and I talked about the struggle to maintain balance in our lives. Dr. Hern frequently travels to South America to do research on native cultures. It is his stress release, along with his writing. He has published articles and books on many topics, including reproductive medicine.

Protesters targeted my friend Liz Karlin after she began her own clinic in Wisconsin. At one point, extremist picketers held a vigil outside her home in Madison. For hours they marched around and around her house. They believed that they could make her walls tumble down by divine intervention, like the walls of Jericho. In her case, it only galvanized neighborhood support for her work.

Every one of us knows that we are likely on a hit list, that we are watched, our families are monitored, and our personal information is circulated by enemies who wish us harm. Being the target of deranged armed fanatics comes with the territory. The fact that self-appointed vigilantes are out to get us, and that we can't always count on protection from our legal, political, and law enforcement agencies, is the harsh, daily price all abortion providers pay to continue working.

I had accepted those terms with eyes wide open. For years I vowed never to bow to the pressure, never to miss a day of clinic due to the protesters. Part of my core resolve was fueled by a stubborn refusal to give the anti-abortion zealots any measure of satisfaction, any claim to bringing my work to a stop.

But was stubbornness enough to keep me going? For me, it no longer had anything to do with threats and intimidation. It wasn't a battle with protesters anymore. I had lost my own clinic. I had spent years shuttling back and forth across the country for work and family. I was exhausted. I was torn. And, while I continued to provide abortions in St. Paul, it was more and more obvious that my employer didn't value my services.

Other people, most people, make job changes. Did I have to keep providing abortions all my professional life? Why shouldn't I explore other possibilities? Why shouldn't I enjoy a more normal existence? I had other interests, other potential—why not?

•

Friday morning. A work day in St. Paul. I was heading into a room to go through the informed consent material with a young patient who did not speak English. One of the staff came with me to serve as a translator.

The patient had been driven almost two hundred miles for this face-to-face appointment necessitated by the language barrier and by the state law mandating that she receive scripted information about abortion twenty-four hours before her procedure. Her abortion was scheduled for the following day, and she would have to make a second round trip for that.

During our stilted conversation, it became clear that, because of an abnormal last menses, she could very possibly be at least a month further along than anticipated, in which case we wouldn't be able to perform her abortion. The best way to verify her status was to do an ultrasound.

Without thinking, I reached up to turn on the ultrasound machine. A staff member in the room interrupted me. "She'll have to pay for that today, you know. If she can't pay, you can't do it."

"Look," I said. "She has traveled almost four hours to get here. She'll do the same tomorrow. She'll be paying for her abortion then, and the cost of the ultrasound is included in her fee."

"I know, but clinic policy is that she has to pay today or wait until tomorrow."

I could feel myself heat up. This sort of bureaucratic nonsense in the face of common sense drives me nuts. I tried to stay calm. "If we wait for the ultrasound, and it turns out she is too far along for us to do the abortion, she'll have to make another eight-hour round trip to a different clinic whenever she can make an appointment there! If we can determine her status right now, using the ultrasound that is a normal part of the abortion procedure, we might save her that trip, not to mention days off work, childcare expenses, and all the anxiety."

I was talking to a wall. The staff person just shook her head.

I excused myself and went to talk to the clinic manager. She was sympathetic but said her hands were tied. Orders from administration, she said. No one was to receive services without paying for it on the spot.

I pleaded, but it got me nowhere. I went to the next level, an administrator who was involved in establishing clinic policies and who happened to be there. I recapped the story, stressed the burden it would place on the patient. "There is no real cost to the clinic to use the ultrasound," I argued. "The machine is right there, and I get paid nothing for doing an ultrasound reading."

"No," she said.

I looked at her for a second; then I lost it. I needed an interpreter to talk to *these* people, not the patient. We had such completely opposed priorities. I couldn't believe they didn't understand the situation and the absurdity of their inflexibility.

"Can't you see what this means for this patient?" I blurted out.

"We simply can't give away services," she repeated.

"I really don't believe anymore that you care as much for the patients as you do for your salary!" I whirled around, slammed the door, and returned to the patient. I'll be the first to admit that the anger I expressed was unprofessional.

Back with the patient, I proceeded to conduct a pelvic exam to help date the pregnancy. It wasn't as good as an ultrasound, but it would give me an approximate time frame.

I was tempted to ignore the administrator and do an ultrasound, but I resisted the impulse.

I hadn't asked permission to do the pelvic exam. I knew full well that it was a service patients would normally be charged for, but I didn't give a damn. I couldn't imagine that they'd fire me for a procedure so clearly in the best interests of a patient.

At the end of the day I left for home in a despondent mood. Several of the staff had come up to me to express their support, but I was butting my head against a wall when it came to the management. I lamented the memory of the clinics I'd worked in fifteen years earlier. Where were people like Maggie Cage and Susan Hill? The warriors who knew that the bottom line was the women we served, not some board of directors riveted to the profit/loss spreadsheet.

I ached for my own clinic, where every staff person had a voice, where no patient was ever turned away for lack of resources, where I could face the trials of each day in solidarity with staff and patients. I drove through the city traffic, into the more rural countryside, seeing nothing, spinning with thoughts and emotions.

On Monday morning the clinic called. One of the administrators was on the line. "Your services are no longer needed," she said, without prelude. "Your contract is terminated, effective immediately."

At first, no one would give me a reason. "We aren't required to give you a reason," they said.

Eventually some vague pretense involving insurance coverage was offered. Everyone knew differently, but I had no recourse. I had worked there for sixteen years, off and on. I had an extremely low complication rate. I had been named the Physician of the Year by the parent organization just four years earlier. I had watched five clinic managers come and go. I had helped fashion clinic protocols and train new staff. Now I'd been fired for putting a patient first.

Within days I was driving west to Montana.

Sonja and I had been in the car together more than four hours. The vehicle dipped and curved along the quiet Montana highway. The spectacular, mountain-rimmed scenery of the Seeley-Swan Valley scrolled past. We talked nonstop, racing from topic to topic, only breaking the flow to exclaim at another incredible view. It was a glorious summer day to spend with my grown-up daughter.

Inevitably, the book I was writing came up. I knew we would come to this, but when we did, I felt my hands grow clammy. I gripped the steering wheel. The mountains blurred.

We had already talked a little about the project. I had told Sonja that there were things revealed that she didn't know about, perhaps some things she would find hard, including a story about Flower Grandma.

"Of course I don't know everything that's gone on all these years," she had said, "but whatever it is about Flower Grandma, I'd like you to tell me first, before I read it."

Now it was time. Briefly, I thought about some way to escape, some way to avoid telling her. I even considered putting the book project on hold, anything to avoid confronting her with this difficult truth about the great-grandmother who had meant Swedish pancakes and fresh cookies and soft, loving hands . . . who had meant everything to Sonja.

"Mom?" Sonja brought me back.

I couldn't get out of this. No escape. Now. I felt the warm tears start down my cheeks. I didn't try to stop them. I knew I couldn't. I took a deep breath, looked straight ahead. I reached over blindly, fumbled for Sonja's hand, squeezed it tight. She squeezed back.

"Sonja. When Flower Grandma was only sixteen, her best friend got pregnant. . . ."

— chapter fourteen

I took refuge in the smell of sage, in the dry winds, in the sharp ridges of the Bridger Mountains, in the home I'd built between Montana mountain ranges. I holed up, lost myself in chores and projects. Whenever my thoughts returned to the shock of losing my job, or to the decisions that would dictate my future, I headed out the door, got my work gloves on, and walked down the dirt road. For entire afternoons I occupied myself making tiles in a neighbor's ceramic studio. Weeks went past in the flurry of distractions and in my determined state of denial. I wasn't ready to cope.

Then, one evening, I was cleaning out a closet when I happened on a box of stuff I hadn't looked at in years. It was jammed with old journals, scrapbooks, letters from patients, news clippings, copies of speeches I'd given. On impulse, I carried the box to the couch under my big window, turned on the lamp, and dove in.

A journal entry nearly a decade old took me back to a dance I'd gone to with a friend in Bozeman one night. We were in a funky bar, dancing to '70s rock 'n' roll tunes. At one point I noticed that my partner had backed away. I looked around. I was encircled by five women. They were smiling at me. Some of them looked familiar. Then the recognition kicked in. They were former patients of mine, women who had come to my clinic. They were paying tribute, dancing with me, around me, locking eyes, saying thanks. None of them said a word. We smiled at each other, danced together through the song, and then they moved off again, back to their partners, their lives.

I pulled out a fat scrapbook compiled by the staff of Mountain Country Women's Clinic, full of patient stories, pictures of the office, news clippings from the Michael Ross trial, a photo of me sitting on the witness stand, testifying. I found myself turning the pages, alternately crying and laughing.

I went through the box but still wasn't satiated. In another container I found my old journals. Every evening for days I returned to them, some of which went back to my medical school training. The emotions and events flowed through me again afresh. I was back with Sonja when she was a toddler, pulling her across campus in a wagon full of books. I was hiding in the guest bedroom at a friend's house because I'd been barricaded from my home by protesters. I was marching at the front of a crowd of a million pro-choice supporters in Washington, DC. I was struggling through the palpable hatred of chanting antis at an airport, holding hands with a woman in that poignant transition after her procedure, coming home to a stranger's muddy bootprints in my apartment, reveling in the exhilarating first days after opening my own clinic.

The immersion in memories made the pain and dislocation of the present shift into perspective. Fortified by the history held in that box, I put out feelers and started to brainstorm possibilities. I began to write again, letting it all out, confused and tangled as it was. I challenged myself to take the advice I'd given to so many patients over the years: it does no good to live by "what if" and "if only."

Not only was it time to move forward, I couldn't afford not to make a move. My finances were dwindling. Bills kept coming. I had to come up with something—and soon. Problem was, I didn't know how.

I volunteered for some community events, gave a talk at a senior center about Alzheimer's disease, joined a group who gave seniors rides to medical appointments, did some housekeeping, and picked up prescriptions. I wasn't getting paid, but I was rejoining the world, meeting people, feeling useful.

I found out about a local women's group in Livingston, Montana. They were dedicated to addressing a broad spectrum of social issues, ranging from education to tolerance. I started going to their meetings and showing up at their activities. Many of the women reinforced my own beliefs and values. I hadn't realized how much I was craving a social and intellectual outlet.

Sometimes we met in someone's home. Twenty or thirty of us would mill around, share a potluck meal, talk. Other times we gathered at the community library to hear a speaker. There was always spirited discussion. I drove home energized, thoughts zipping along, feeling empowered by the solidarity and compassion in the group.

At one meeting a woman came up behind me and took my arm. "Susan," she said, "where are you working these days?" I'd known her for some time and had heard that she'd taken the job of medical director for an organization that ran a number of clinics in Montana.

"Ah, well," I stammered. "Not really anywhere. I'm sort of between things."

"Would you consider working for us?" she asked.

I felt my pulse pick up. I almost said yes before she finished the question, but I caught myself.

"Tell me more," I said, a guarded tone in my voice.

"Well, there's not much to tell," she said. "We have several clinics widely scattered across the state. We're losing one of our providers. I was hoping you might be willing to help us out."

It wasn't until that moment, when the real prospect of going back to work was laid before me, that I realized how much I'd missed the contact with patients and the rewards of my work. It had been my professional life for more than two decades. My time away from it had only fed my passion for that work. By the same token, I'd been deeply hurt and disappointed by an organization that, in my experience, often prioritized billing protocol over patient well-being. I couldn't afford to be naïve, and I was wary about opening that door again so soon.

"I'll be honest with you," I said. "It's very appealing. I love the work, and I think I'm good at what I do. But I have concerns. I can't commit to anything before those concerns are addressed."

"Here's my phone number," she said, handing me her card. "Please do call."

The next day I did, in spite of myself. I couldn't stand the suspense. I told her about my experiences in Minnesota and my fears of finding myself in similar situations. She forwarded me to the organization CEO and the clinical services manager. I told them straight out that I was not simply a technician paid to conduct procedures. We talked about the importance of counseling, of responding to each patient's needs and circumstances, of putting patients ahead of strict policies and rules.

I tried to read between the lines of their responses, get an intuitive sense for their attitudes and tendencies. I put them on the spot with specific patient scenarios that might butt up against clinic regulations. What about women who don't have the full fee? I asked. What about providing an extra service to an indigent patient to save her another trip to the clinic? What about allowing a family member or friend into the procedure room if it soothes the patient?

At the end of the phone conversations, I felt reassured enough to give it a trial run. "Let's see how it goes for a time or two," I said. "I can't commit beyond that until I get a feel for how this will all work."

Within a month I was making my first commute, a two-hour drive to Helena, Montana. The miles slipped past, full of sky and river valley scenery. I knew full well that if this experience didn't work out, it might signal the end of my career with women's clinics. I wanted so badly for things to go well, to return to the nurturing atmosphere I'd known in years past.

I had been to the Helena clinic before, even worked a few days there half a dozen years ago. I had memories of a place full of warmth and compassion, but that had been then. No doubt much had changed, including the administration.

I was early. I stopped for a cup of coffee, knowing it was a procrastination device. I pressed my head against the steering wheel, tried to calm myself. I was hopeful, eager, nervous, and scared stiff.

I still wasn't ready when I pulled in to the parking lot behind the clinic, but I fought down the impulse to turn around and drive back home. I forced myself out of the car, grabbed my bag, walked to the door. Just another day of work, I told myself. Don't make it more than it is.

Familiar faces greeted me, staff who had been there for years. I was pulled into hugs. "It's good to see you again! Thanks so much for coming all this way."

I took a deep breath, looked around. Very little had changed. I remembered the cubbyholes full of information and brochures on family planning, IUDs, sexually transmitted diseases, how to talk about sex, Pap smears. The furnishings were well-worn but comfortable and inviting.

I went to change into my scrubs, passing one of the staff with a patient along the way.

"Here, this will warm you up a bit," I overheard the nurse saying in a soft voice as she wrapped a blanket around the woman's shoulders.

My fears began to fade. Everything was so familiar—and so new. A fresh start for me, but the same decisions being made, the same fears being faced, the same questions in patients' eyes. The same tension and fear faced by thousands of women every year. It is the farthest thing from mundane for each patient on this day, at this clinic.

As the hours passed, my confidence and optimism grew. I was back in my element. Everything I saw, and more importantly, my intuitive reading of things, gave me hope that this organization truly did its best to put patients first. The staff was efficient, cheerful, respectful. Opinions were offered and honored. When a protocol came into question, the administration and staff worked together to find a solution. I didn't pick up any underlying tension or resentment between management and staff.

By the end of the day the job counseling I'd received, the other lines of work I'd explored, the doubts I had about continuing my clinic work had vanished. This was where I belonged. This was what I did best. This was where I felt fulfilled and valuable.

Before leaving for home, I met briefly with the staff. None of them had any idea how vulnerable and shaky I'd felt when I walked through the door that morning or how tentative I'd been about my future.

"Thank you," I said. "Thanks to all of you." I didn't know how to capture my feelings. I felt tears welling up. "Thank you for caring about these women and for being here."

"Of course we care," one of them said. "Why else would we work here?"

"But," I struggled to compose myself, "it's so much more than that. This isn't just a job for any of you. You're all skilled and professional, but you're more than that. You're compassionate. You're dedicated. I don't think you know how much that means to every patient who comes here—and to me, especially today." I broke off. "It is such a relief," I finally blurted out, laughing through tears.

Over the next months I began working at several clinics around the state. These are places that are only open one day every two weeks. Just two days a month. Many patients wait two to four weeks for an appointment and then drive as many as six hours to get there. As the physician I drive up to seven hours to get to work. Montana is big country, and women come from all over the region, including Canada.

I settled into the routine, such as it was. Patients came and went, each unique, but some more memorable than others.

"Dr. Wicklund, would you please look at this ultra-sound?" one of the clinic staff asked me.

"From the looks of it, the measurements put her at the edge of my limit," I observed, after looking at the image. "Is it her first pregnancy? Maybe we should send her to Billings."

"You might need to hear the rest of her story," the nurse said.

We sat down.

"This patient is nineteen years old. And yes, it is her first pregnancy. It was extremely hard for her to get here today. Going to Billings in a week may as well be the moon. Worse than that, she told me she knows someone on the reservation who will do the abortion for her. She is absolutely serious. If we send her away, that's her next option."

These revelations never fail to stun me. I have seen the women with scarred, torn cervical tissue, with lacerations, women who have been mutilated out of desperation. But it still seems so primitive, so barbaric that I tend to bury the reality until it confronts me again. In our modern, sophisticated, medically advanced country, women are still using coat hangers and sticks and toxic concoctions to end unwanted pregnancies. No one truly knows how common it is now. There are no statistics. What is clear is that if the anti-choice forces have their way, it will become prevalent again.

"Okay," I said. "I better go see her."

"Hi, I'm Dr. Wicklund. You can call me Sue. How are you doing?"

"Oh, I'm fine. Really. They already warned me that you might not be willing to do the abortion today." She was not wringing her hands. There was no pleading tone in her voice.

Perhaps she's not so sure about her decision as we suspect, I thought. Maybe she was just exploring an option, and now she has an excuse not to do it. "Are you sure you want to end this pregnancy?" I asked her.

"Oh yes." She looked me in the eye. "I have no intention of continuing this pregnancy. No way. But my friend can do it for me. She offered to do it in the first place. She's done lots of them before, on herself and other girls, but I thought it might be better to come here first. Listen, if you can't do it, it's okay. I know she can." Her confidence was chilling. This young girl was so naïve, it took my breath away.

"Don't you understand that you could die having an abortion like that?" I asked her, gently.

"Oh no, you don't understand. My friend knows what she's doing."

I sighed. We talked about other things—her plans to get an education beyond high school, her siblings who had dropped out of school, her steady job. I talked about the time I spent on public assistance and how I decided to be a doctor even though I had a young child.

It was very clear, at the end of our conversation, that if she left without having her abortion, she'd have her friend perform an illegal and dangerous one.

I had her lie down so I could examine her cervix. I was re-assured to find that it had already softened up, which re-duced the chance for any complications. I looked at the young woman on the exam table. I thought about her life and this crossroads. I stood up.

"We'll proceed," I said.

Her abortion was safe and routine. I knew that she would be able to have children some day, if and when she was ready.

"Listen," I said to her before she left. "Here's my phone number. I want you to tell your friend to call me. I'm not try-ing to get her in trouble. I want to see what we can do to help women in your community. And I want to ask her how she does her abortions. Maybe I'll be able to share some sto-ries with her."

"Sure," she said. "I believe you."

I never did hear from her friend.

Outside the clinics, the protesters gather. They hold signs; they say prayers; they call out to women coming for an appointment. Much of the time, the homegrown protesters are relatively peaceful and unthreatening. They come out of conviction, out of strongly held moral beliefs. I can respect that. As long as they don't infringe on the rights of others, they have as much right to free speech and demonstration as any American.

Over the years I have even had conversations with several protesters. To tell the truth, I want to know where they're coming from, what their true objectives are.

When I was working in the Midwest, one young protester followed me everywhere. Once, in a grocery store, I came around the end of an aisle, and we came face to face. We stood perfectly still. I looked hard at him.

"So, instead of following me around all the time and trying to intimidate me, why don't you come have a cup of coffee?" I asked. I was as surprised at my words as he was.

He stared at me. "N-no, no, I don't think so," he stammered. But he didn't turn to go.

"Why not?" I continued, emboldened. "I want to hear what you have to say. You can't possibly think I'd hurt you, do you? Why follow me around if you're afraid to even talk to me?"

He thought for a minute. I had him cornered. "Well, okay," he said. "I'll meet you at the coffee shop in twenty minutes." He turned and walked quickly away.

I didn't know whether to believe him, but twenty minutes later we faced each other across a table.

"Why do you follow me everywhere?" I asked.

"I want you to stop killing babies," he said.

"Oh come on. You can do better than that. Why don't you tell me what you know about abortion?"

"I know it's dangerous," he said. "I know women are scarred for life, physically and emotionally."

"I wish you'd do some reading on your own rather than just believe what the other protesters tell you. Abortion is the safest minor surgery performed in the United States. Women are not scarred from it."

I wrote down some references for him to look up, including government publications. I walked him through the procedure. "Even though it's classified as minor surgery, there is nothing sharp, no cutting instruments, no stitches, no scalpels."

I could tell he was shocked. He'd been immersed in the rhetoric of the antis, where knives and scalpels killed babies and maimed women. "But you are taking a human life," he argued. "You are a murderer."

"Would you really call me a killer?" I asked him, point blank.

"Yes, I would. It's a human life you are taking. I don't know what else to call you."

I thought of the small sac and villi I remove in an abortion procedure, tissue that has no capacity to feel pain, think, or have any sense of being. To people like this young man, that tiny sac is a human being.

To me, that tissue represents potential, and the woman carrying it has to have the freedom and ability to nurture and grow that potential. Not every seed that falls from a pinecone becomes a tree. The soil has to be fertile; the climate and topography and timing have to be favorable. If those ingredients are wrong, that potential growth never takes place.

For the black-and-white protesters, women are reduced to little more than incubators. Their role is to produce babies, no matter what the circumstances. Where do their rights, their pursuit of happiness, their ambitions enter the equation? Why, like for the seed that falls, aren't the conditions for growth considered?

We talked for more than an hour. I gained respect for his convictions and earnest beliefs. He, I think, learned a few things about the realities of abortion and the tough life dilemmas women are faced with.

Several times over the ensuing months we met and talked more. The last time we spoke was just before he was entering a seminary. At the end of the conversation, before we parted ways, he said, "You know, I can't hate you any more."

I don't know what happened to him after that, but I never again saw him protesting outside of a clinic.

The professional protesters are the ones I fear. They are mostly men, and for them, protesting is a full-time obsession. They target different regions in the country or particularly vulnerable clinics. They bring their hate-filled slogans, their planes that fly over towns and cities pulling banners depicting bloody babies, their confrontational tactics. When they come to town, I wear my bulletproof vest and carry my gun. Unfortunately, their views have infiltrated the laws and policies of our country and the lives of my patients.

•

"Pleased to meet you, ma'am," the young woman said, after I introduced myself.

She was a Montana resident and member of the military stationed in Germany.

"How long are you home for?" I asked.

"Just long enough to get this abortion, a note from you that I'm no longer pregnant, and then I'm on a plane headed back to Germany."

"Are you telling me that you had to come all the way back here to have an abortion?"

She nodded. "Our government won't allow abortions in military facilities, so this was my only option. I had to leave my unit for almost a week and pay my own way to fly from Germany to Montana so I could continue to serve my country. Seems pretty stupid, doesn't it? Here we are, overseas, fighting for other people's freedom, but mine is taken away."

It isn't only the United States military that marches to the anti-abortion drumbeat, but all recipients of our foreign aid. In Africa and Asia and throughout the developing world, humanitarian aid is cut off if family planning counseling includes any discussion of abortion, or if women are referred to clinics that provide abortion services. If the option of abortion appears anywhere on the radar, it negates aid for well-baby care, infant formula, prenatal care, HIV treatment and counseling, and a host of other critically important medical services.

Worldwide, more than five hundred thousand women die each year from complications during pregnancy and childbirth. Tens of thousands of those deaths could be prevented by reproductive health care provided in clinics, the same care often denied because of the gag rule. Clinics in the United States are also cut off from federal funding and aid if abortion appears in the repertoire of services.

Sometimes the "gags" have nothing to do with the government or political atmosphere, but are self-imposed: silence and hypocritical denial enforced by the fear of public exposure.

One day in Kalispell, Montana, I stood before another young woman. She had her head down, wouldn't look at me. Staff had warned me that she seemed repressed and unresponsive. They hoped I'd be able to get her to open up.

"Ruth," I insisted. "We're concerned about what's pushing you to make this decision. We need to be sure this is something you decide for yourself, not for anyone else. I need you to tell me if you really and truly want this abortion."

"Yes, I do," she said quietly, still not looking up. "I want to finish college."

"I was a single mom through college and medical school," I told her. "It's not impossible."

She didn't respond.

"I'm not trying to talk you out of an abortion, but I'm getting the feeling that there is more to this than going to school. If you won't tell me what's going on, I can't proceed with an abortion."

She finally lifted her head. Her eyes met mine, held mine, seemed to assess me. She sighed.

"My parents are very religious," she began. "My dad is a deacon at the church. If I have a baby out of wedlock, it would be a mark on them. It would say to all their friends that their daughter has sinned. Sex out of marriage. It's a terrible sin, and it would make them look bad."

"Okay, so you've sinned in their eyes, but how do they feel about abortion?" I asked.

She laughed bitterly. "Oh, abortion. That's totally unforgivable. But it's the lesser evil because it would be a secret. If I have an abortion, their friends in church will never know."

"So you're having an abortion to protect them?"

"No, I'm having an abortion so I can finish college."

I looked at her, my face full of questions. The clock hummed on the wall.

"This is the situation," she went on. "I live at home. My folks help pay my college tuition. Their income is high enough that I would never qualify for student grants, and they won't cosign on a student loan. If I have this baby, they will kick me out of the house and take away any financial help. I would be banned from my family."

"They have TOLD you this?" I couldn't keep the outrage out of my voice.

"In no uncertain terms," she nodded.

"Well, that's certainly a Christian thing to do . . ." I caught myself too late. The words were out. I usually enforce strict neutrality on my interactions with patients, even if I am shocked and appalled by a statement. I bite my tongue a lot, but this time I slipped up. I felt my face go red with embarrassment, but when I looked at Ruth, she was just nodding sadly in agreement.

Sometimes, when I catch myself judging others, I circle around and look at myself, the paths I've taken and the prices I've paid. I don't spend a lot of time regretting things, but if I'm honest, I have to recognize the truth. My commitments have demanded a great deal from the people I love.

Sonja is thirty years old now. She is one of the most kind, loving, competent young women I know. I am immensely proud of her. But I can't escape the pangs of guilt I feel for the years I was absent, the things I missed doing with her. For much of her youth, Randy might as well have been a single parent. I worked one hundred hours a week, missed parent-teacher conferences, missed doing homework together, going to swim meets, helping Sonja through tough times with friends. Randy, and sometimes David, her stepdad and dad went to the conferences, stood on the sidelines at games. They were there together often enough that some of Sonja's classmates thought she had gay parents.

Those two men picked up the loose ends, they covered for me, and Sonja persevered and triumphed in spite of the challenges I threw her way. I know that my marriages, and to some extent, my relationship with my daughter, have suffered because of my commitments.

It continues to this day, that compromise. Julie is still back in Wisconsin dealing with Dad. Her life is bound up with his care every day. I am involved with his medical treatment. I take care of his finances. We've been able to keep him living at home, the house he's lived in more than fifty years. I have made the two-thousand-mile round-trip drive from Montana to Wisconsin more times than I can count, in response to every imaginable emergency, but I have also chosen to carry on with my life.

Recently I drove to my family home again, across the plains of eastern Montana, through the badlands of North Dakota, into the forests and fields and humidity of the Midwest. At the end, weary with highway hours, I pulled in to the same leaf-strewn driveway where I learned to ride a bike, where I set up hay bales to practice parallel parking, where I galloped on horseback, my hair flying.

Flower Grandma's trailer had been pulled away years earlier, replaced by a poorly tended garden. The house needed paint. The bird feeder hung broken and empty. But the creek still whispered below the house. When I stepped out of the car, I heard the wind in the white pines, the sound that strips away the decades and makes me a young girl.

"Hi Dad!" I strode up the steps to the door. I knew his hearing aid was likely missing or turned off.

"Dad! It's Sue. I'm home from Montana for a visit."

He looked at me blankly, and then recognition fired up his eyes. He opened his arms wide to hug me.

"Hey, maybe we should go somewhere," he said. He didn't ask how I was, what my drive was like. I was a possibility for escape.

"I thought maybe I could beat you in a game of cribbage," I offered, instead.

"Yep, by golly. Let's do that."

But we couldn't find the cards. He had moved them from the cupboard where they'd been for forty years. Looking around the living room I saw a note in Dad's writing taped to the television. "You people get out of here and quit using my electricity!"

Julie had told me he talks to people on the TV, waves to them. He sees himself in the mirror and thinks that it's his brother, Elmer. He's convinced that Elmer lives with him, but he gets frustrated with him because he won't answer.

"Someone came in here and stole those cards." Dad was getting upset. I tried to push us into another direction, to change the mood. Finally, he turned to me. "Vera," he said, "let's have coffee."

"That sounds good," I said. I thought of Mom, her name hanging in the air, and of her life energy that I still felt in the house. I poured a dose of that Scandinavian liquid magic into our cups and sat down across from Dad, wondering whom he saw facing him.

Four days in Wisconsin, tending to some medication details, catching up with Julie, shouldering the load of Dad's care briefly, then back to Montana in time for a Mother's Day peace rally I'd helped coordinate.

For months we had been making calls, sending emails, printing posters, organizing interviews, gathering support from around the state. Many other organizations joined up.

Speakers were coming from around the country. We had music scheduled and expected a huge turnout for our march down the Main Street of Bozeman.

On Sunday morning we were there early, setting up tables, water stations, information booths. The stage and sound system went up, along with the children's tent. Ready to go. Great energy from everyone.

My cell phone rang. It was Julie.

"Just wanted to wish you luck today, Sis."

"Thanks," I said. "How's Dad?"

"Oh, you know. Same old, same old. We're taking him on a picnic to the lake today."

"Have fun," I said.

A pause.

"Hey, Julie?" I continued.

"What?"

"Thanks for being there."

I closed the phone, started up the entrance road toward the stage. People were streaming in to the rally. Families, old people, kids in strollers, couples with picnic blankets, people carrying handmade signs and posters about peace. Hundreds of people.

I noticed a truck pulled up to the curb, someone erecting large signs on the back. Bloody pictures. Dead babies. Anti-abortion rhetoric. All the good energy I'd been feeling drained away, along with my feelings of well-being and hope. I stopped, stunned by the awful contrast, stricken by the old knot of fear.

"Susan Wicklund!" A rough man's voice shouting from near the truck. A man pointing at me. "Susan Wicklund! Stop killing babies. Stop the murder!"

People turned to look at me. Instinctively, I wheeled away and started walking fast. I wouldn't look back, but I felt like a target, waited for the sound of a shot. I reached for my left side, where I would sometimes carry the .38 Special. Not there. I hadn't worn the gun in months. A decrease in clinic violence had lulled me into believing that I had a normal life. I pulled out the walkie-talkie and paged one of the rally organizers.

"Margie," I said, urgently, "the antis are here. They have identified me. They're putting up signs and—"

"Get out of there right now," her voice cut me off. "Go to the area behind the stage and stay there. Go now! You have to stay out of sight."

Crestfallen, I followed directions. I knew she was right. The old brew of emotions rose in me like bile, bitter and angry. That old dread that used to boil up every time I turned the car key in the ignition, every time the phone rang, every time I stepped off of a plane. Damn! Why today?!

In the area behind the stage, though, it felt comfortable, protected. There were details I could help with, questions I could answer. I saw people I knew. We waved to each other. I ignored the bad taste of confrontation, regained some of my positive momentum.

"Sue, are you okay?" Margie popped in to check on me. "We're about to start."

"Yes, I'm fine," I told her. "Let's make this a great day."

"Listen," Margie continued. "Would you mind sitting with Elsie Fox? We'll be bringing her on stage in a bit. I think you'd enjoy talking with her."

Elsie was ninety-eight years old. She had been an activist all her adult life. She was a veteran of civil rights marches, nonviolent demonstrations, labor rallies in San Francisco, causes and events that stretched back before the Depression. She had lived through both world wars, rode in horse-drawn buggies, could remember when women first got to vote.

She was sitting quietly backstage in a chair in the shade of a tree. I walked over to her and introduced myself. She wore a straw hat that covered white curls of hair. A colorful string of beads hung around her neck. She wore sunglasses, red lipstick. She could have been anyone's grandmother, or great-grandmother, for that matter.

She looked at me with a clear, discerning gaze. Her hands were clasped loosely in her lap, holding down a sheaf of papers, her speech. I had heard from friends that she had been practicing for weeks.

"Susan," she said. "That was your name, wasn't it?"

"Yes," I moved closer. "We've spoken on the phone before. It's so good to put a face with a name."

"Susan," she repeated. She turned to face me. "Tell me what you do."

I hesitated. Should I tell her the truth or gloss over it? I didn't want to distract her with other thoughts before she got up in front of the crowd. I didn't want to face her reaction if she didn't approve. I pulled over a crate and sat down close beside her. Nearby people scurried past, oblivious to the two women behind the stage. A jungle of cords and speaker wires surrounded us.

"I am a doctor," I began. "I have been providing safe, legal abortions for women for nearly twenty years."

A long silence. The sound of the crowd faded in the intensity of our focus. Elsie turned her face away, her gaze fixed in the distance. She stayed very still. I didn't dare move or speak. Enough time passed that I wondered if she'd heard me. Or was she reworking her own memories? Perhaps she was measuring her response. Then she shifted, seemed to sit taller in her chair.

Her hand reached out and found mine. She pulled my hand to the arm of her chair, covered it with hers. Her soft, old hand gently patted mine.

"That's good," she said. "That's real good."

— epilogue

Thank goodness I liked this book—that was my first reaction. If I hadn't, no amount of faint praise would have convinced my mother that I did. I've never been able to lie, especially to her. And she's never lied to me, except for my own safety. But she did hide things from me, it turns out.

It's not that I was unaware of the events or facts about which you have just read, with the exception of Flower Grandma's tragic secret. Growing up, I knew what my mother did for a living. I knew the moral questions raised by abortion. I heard many of the patients' stories, and I knew about the abortion early in Mom's life that inspired her convictions. I was well aware of the protesters and the death threats, the arson attempts and stalkings.

I also knew that Mom was on the front lines defending a new and still-fragile women's right—that she was and is one of the brave few who live out their convictions through action.

What I did not know was the depth of her fear and uncertainty. I believed that through it all she was as strong as she pretended to be when I was around, as casual about the sacrifices as she always led me to believe. The disguises? I thought they were fun, and she played along. The midnight drives to Fargo? I thought she just didn't like flying in small planes. The days when the protesters were thick as flies? She and I relived the humorous stories, like when a neighbor removed the muffler from his riding lawn mower, began to mow his lawn, and then left the machine running in the corner of his yard, right next to the protesters. He claimed the engine overheated.

It turns out that Mom made a point of collecting herself, planning her words and approach, before telling me things. That was the hardest part of reading this book: accepting the emotional turmoil of the person who was my model of strength and courage.

Over the past year, I have repeatedly discussed passages with her: "Did you really think you weren't smart enough to be a doctor? . . . You couldn't have been that scared to tell Flower Grandma about your work. . . . How come I didn't realize you felt so unsafe, even inside the clinics? . . . Why were you so nervous about going back to work in Montana?" Mom's fear of protesters was natural, but I never imagined that she doubted her path and had moments when she considered giving up her work. I have even more respect for her now that I know.

Facing Mom's demons as I read the book naturally led me to relive my own fears, such as a vivid nightmare from the very early years: crowds of people in front of the Fargo clinic, parting neatly for Mom until one man with a gun, in slow motion, steps out, shoves aside the security escort, shoots her three times while camera bulbs flash. I woke screaming. I was fourteen years old, shocked by the image of my mother lying in a pool of her own blood. Mom ran into my bedroom to comfort me, assured me that it was just a dream.

The anti-choice activists were picketing the clinics and our home at that time, following her to work, trying to shame our family, intimidate our friends, but they wouldn't kill someone. They wouldn't go that far, she said.

Of course, they did go that far, more than once, and I fell apart whenever a shooting occurred. I would feel the ground shift under me when I heard the news, find my way dizzily home, and cry for hours, curled up on my bed, so shocked by every new act of violence. I was devastated for the victims and their families, of course, but it was the fear we would be next that paralyzed me.

The harassment, the "wanted" posters, the crowds of protesters during high school—they were all stressful, but I had an excellent network of family, friends, teachers, and neighbors who protected and reassured me. Even the local Baptist minister encouraged his largely anti-choice congregation to come to our aid. In a way, the public harassment and the incredibly supportive reaction of our community just proved to me that people are overwhelmingly good, kind, and caring. My only real fear was that an act of violence might claim Mom. The possibility terrified me. I didn't want to be the weak link, though. I knew that I was the only person in the world who could actually convince her to quit her job, but I also knew that I could be strong and play my small part by standing up to the pressure.

Yet just this year, I insisted that I had no lasting trauma from those times.

"Surely it still affects you, at least a little?" Mom's coauthor, Al, asked me as we sat discussing the soon-to-be-published book after dinner one evening. I considered his question. It was the middle of a vacation from my teaching job. Mom and I had spent the day running errands, talking nonstop about the usual—the antics of our neighbors, my graduate school applications, a cousin's new baby, upcoming camping trips.

"Our lives are not extraordinary," I insisted. "I hardly think of the times when the protesters were really after us."

"Nothing has stuck with you from those experiences?" Al asked again.

And then I remembered. I had glanced into the back seat while slamming the car door on one of our many stops that day.

"Mom," I yelled as she walked toward the store, "unlock the car—the mail is face up, and I can read your name."

Never leave names or personal information visible through a window: just one of a hundred permanently ingrained security routines. I turned the mail face down and went inside. I guess a baseline of fear will always be present.

This book has refreshed good memories along with the bad, especially of holidays and summers spent in Montana. In the winter, I brought friends with me, and we went skiing up in the mountains. In the summer, Mom took long weekends off, and she and I hiked, rode horses, and canoed the Yellowstone River. During the week, between babysitting jobs and going to the swimming pool, I loved to stop by the clinic. I said hi to the staff, made sure Mom ate lunch, read the myriad thank-you cards from patients (with names blacked out, of course), and witnessed the care taken with each woman's physical and emotional well-being, from reception area to recovery room.

Once, a patient granted permission for me to watch her abortion. I was curious and needed to know firsthand that the horrible bloody-baby posters carried by the protesters were a lie. The procedure was just as Mom had always described it—quick and anticlimactic, producing a small amount of cloudy-looking tissue and a visibly relieved woman. I remember wishing I could take each protester one by one with me on these visits. I was convinced that a day in the clinic, hearing the honest dialogue with patients, witnessing the reality of an abortion procedure, would help them thoughtfully reconsider their beliefs and actions.

Or maybe the anti-choice protesters could just ask questions within their own families and then listen carefully to their mothers, grandmothers, sisters, wives, and daughters. It's taboo in our society to discuss abortion on anything less than a political level, but I know the truth. Someone close to each and every one of us has had an abortion. The experience is common, but I do not believe it is taken lightly. Women who have exercised their right to choose never forget.

Hardly a day goes by without a woman greeting Mom warmly in a store, at the gym, or on the street. A shy hello or meaningful squeeze of the hand accompanies looks and words of sincere appreciation and warmth. These women are former patients, representatives of the millions of American women who have an abortion at some point in their lives. They are forever grateful to the loving doctor who helped them see their difficult decision through with dignity.

That doctor is my mother.

Sonja Lynne Wicklund

— afterword

This Common Secret began at my kitchen table more than a decade ago. During the year that Sue lived with my family, staying in a basement room of our small house in Montana, she shared a great many stories. Incredible tales. On Saturday mornings over coffee, or late at night after a long day, Marypat and I would sit and listen to Sue talk.

At some point I said, "Sue, we have to write some of this stuff down."

"I've been thinking about that," she said. "But I'm not a writer, and I've never found the time."

"Well, I'm a writer," I said, "and these stories are important."

When we began our collaboration, we would sit in the living room after the kids went to bed. Sue curled up in a big reading chair, wrapped herself in a blanket, and started talking while I scribbled in pencil on yellow legal pads as fast as I could. Sometimes Sue would shake with the emotion as her stories poured out. Later we met at a local coffee shop, where we worked for hours at a round table. Sue reeled off patient situations, protester confrontations, legal quagmires, counseling scenarios, personal turning points. It was exhausting—and amazing.

For her, it was a way to reckon with the emotional toll, work through her feelings, and record events. For me, the accounts were intense, vivid, and revealing. Sue's memory for detail and her simple, authentic presentation made the writing job easy.

Almost always, at some point in the telling, there were tears. More than once we had to take a break to regain our composure, get another cup of coffee, before we could carry on.

"This is not about me," Sue insisted, from the beginning. "I want this to be about the women, not about me."

I honored her sentiment, knew it was genuine, but I also knew she was wrong. Of course it is about the women she has seen over the years, all of them: their symbolic dilemmas and dramatic situations, what they represent in the larger debate. It is about Flower Grandma, Martina Greywind, the fourteen-year-old victim of incest, the young woman raped on the way home from a movie. But all of that hangs on the framework of Sue's tale—her commitment, her stubborn allegiance, her sense of morality, and her fortitude—beginning with the choice to go to medical school and continuing to this day in her career as an abortion provider.

"I understand, Sue," I said, "and I respect you for it. But this stuff is only a collage of disconnected snapshots without your story."

"I don't want the women to get lost," she insisted.

Sue is a big-boned, straightforward woman with a hearty laugh. She has a rural sense of etiquette, a spontaneous flair for fun, and genuine warmth. Meeting her on the street, you'd never think of her as a warrior. You wouldn't expect her to be controversial in any way. Rather, she is engaging, intelligent, humorous, open-minded, strong-willed. She could be a rancher or teacher or veterinarian.

The fact that Sue is a warrior is a matter of circumstance, not of intention. She is a woman who has followed her heart, who has not been swayed by intimidation or difficulty. In her case, that course has led straight into a firestorm of controversy and danger.

Sitting at our kitchen table over the course of that year, Marypat and I were educated. Like most people, we'd had our experiences with pregnancy decisions. Like most people, we thought we knew the issues and the politics and where we stood. It turned out that, in fact, we had no idea. The power of this project, and the potential impact on readers, is that many will turn the first page thinking that they understand the parameters of the abortion issue in America. They will be floored, as I was.

Having Sue in our home gave us a hint of the wary tension she maintains as a matter of course. I have no doubt that the antis figured out where she'd moved within weeks. I also assumed, perhaps naïvely, that they would never attack her in the midst of a family with young children, that our home offered her the immunity of our embrace.

Her security escort would pull in to our driveway every morning and drop her off again after work. The phone rang at all hours. We had more than the usual number of disconnected calls, sometimes in the dead of night. Some of them were sinister. The presence of someone on the other end was palpable—you could even hear the breathing—then the line would go dead. I found myself scrutinizing people walking past on the sidewalk, taking note if a car slowed down as it drove by our house. When Sue says she knows what it's like to be prey, I have a faint inkling of how that feels.

Sue became, and remains, a fast family friend. We have come to know Sonja. My family has gone on backcountry hikes, horse rides, and canoe trips with Sue and Sonja. Sue assisted in the home birth of our daughter, Ruby. She has been involved in our family life since 1993. Sue sees us regularly when she comes to town, catches up with the kids, shares a meal. She takes care of our dog when we travel.

Initially, when we began writing together, we hoped only to take care of the outpouring, hang on to the immediacy of events. Inevitably, though, the possibility of putting together a book came up. Sue was very nervous about the prospect. It is a subject so prone to sensation. She saw the potential for her tale to spin out of control on the public stage, and it scared the hell out of her. She lives on the hot seat daily; why go public with it and create the potential for more vulnerability and controversy? Why become more of a target than she already is? These are not trivial or overblown concerns.

We worked on the collection of pieces for months, passing them back and forth, kneading them into shape. Eventually we accumulated a manuscript that filled a large file folder. Then we put it away. Years passed. Sue had to close her Bozeman clinic and move back to Wisconsin, where she spent long years caring for her parents.

We visited her in the Midwest, helped her family tap maple trees for syrup, stayed with her relatives, played cribbage with her ailing father, and visited her mother, Vera, in the nursing home just months before she died.

Then, during the fall of 2005, Sue and I met for coffee after a long break. She was back in Montana full-time but was going through a period of transition, considering options. We talked for some time about her uncertain future.

"You know," I said, "I still have that folder full of stories we wrote together."

"I was just looking at my copy of that the other week," Sue said.

"If you ever want to reconsider a book project, I'm game," I said.

"Really!" Sue leaned forward. "It's exactly what I've been thinking. I am finally ready to share those stories. I'm not afraid anymore, or at least I'm not going to give in to fear, and I'm truly fed up with the political debate. In fact, I'm terrified of what's coming down the road for women in this country. We could lose everything we've worked for and return to the time of back-alley abortions."

"Are you sure?"

"Absolutely," Sue said. "I'd start tomorrow. When can we meet?"

As it happens, quite a number of those kitchen table and coffee shop stories made their way into this book. A great many more did not. At some point I had to tell Sue to stop. There was so much, and more all the time. Even as we wrote the final chapters, Sue would arrive with fresh accounts—a woman essentially in a state of bondage who had to escape from her controlling husband long enough to get an abortion, Native American women coping with Third World conditions, or young, fragile victims of incest.

"We're done, Sue," I said. "There's no end. At some point we have to stop."

Alan S. Kesselheim
Bozeman, Montana

— acknowledgments

This book would still be an idea stuck in a backwater were it not for my good friend Alan Kesselheim. In addition to being an established author, Al is passionate about life, family, and the human condition. As coauthor of this book, he kept me moving forward, pushed without nagging, humored my words, and believed it could happen. Al has a gift for listening and then understanding the things not said. More important, he gets to the bottom of the story, drawing it out and making it sing. I cannot thank him enough. His wife, Marypat Zitzer, and their three children, Eli, Sawyer, and Ruby, are family.

Our agent, Kris Dahl with International Creative Management, was brave enough to take this on, for which we are very grateful. Thank you, Maryanne Vollers, for being the bridge.

Some projects are more of a challenge than others, and we are honored that Lisa Kaufman and Susan Weinberg at PublicAffairs recognized the importance of this story and were willing to jump in with such a solid commitment. Our astute editor, Lindsay Jones, was able to convince me to tell more of my personal story. It is clear to us that her editorial guidance made the book stronger.

We are also indebted to a number of information resources for the factual and statistical background used throughout the book. A list of those sources can be found in the Appendix.

There were many friends and colleagues who read various drafts and offered suggestions, comments, and insights. Thanks especially to Velma McMeekin, Maryanne Vollers, Margot Kidder, and Eleanor Smeal. Your enthusiasm, encouragement, and feedback were always well timed.

Throughout my training and for the past twenty years of working in the clinics, I have come to know, love, and respect some incredible people. I am grateful for the things they have taught me, for the personal stories they have shared, and for embracing me as a colleague. Mostly I appreciate their respect for the patients. Thank you Susan Hill, Maggie Cage, Dr. Elizabeth Newhall, Tom Weber, Becky Howell, Kathy, Debbie, Karen, Dottie, Shari, Kathryn, and Judy. A heartfelt thanks, and a promise never to forget, two women now gone: Dr. Elizabeth Karlin and Dr. Jane Hodgson. You are terribly missed.

The six core staff members who worked with me in Bozeman were dedicated, skilled, compassionate, and understanding team members. Together we provided truly exceptional women's reproductive health care. Thanks to Stacey, Kate, Diane, Deb, Kristi, and Holly.

I wish with all my heart that my mother was still alive and could hold this book in her hands. She had a tremendous impact on my life. She was a feminist and social activist in her own right, and she believed this book would happen someday. She was always right. And I hope that some part of my father can understand what this is all about and how much I love him.

When it comes to family, however, my sister, Julie, is the one who has always forgiven me when I suddenly changed course. She listens to my uncertainty and fear, remains calm when I need a rock to rest on, and holds the boat steady while I climb in. Most important, she lets me head downstream without piling on the guilt. Thank you so very much, Julie.

For reasons you each know, thank you to David, Randy, and Rod. You've kept me afloat over a very long journey.

In this past year of sitting up late at the computer, searching for words, trying to find my voice, quietly reliving so many challenging times, I leaned on my best friends, Ben and Steve. They could always recognize when I needed a good meal instead of another bowl of cereal. In between times, I had the guidance of Brad, helping me reclaim my strength in so many ways. Many thanks to you.

Finally, the one person who could have reined me in, the young woman the anti-choice forces failed to break, the kind, strong person who still loves me after all I have put her through: my daughter, Sonja. Her strength and love continue to ground me.

— appendix:
further information
and factual resources

I hope my story does not suggest that anti-abortion activities nationwide have decreased. To the contrary—emboldened by changes in the U.S. Supreme Court and able to recruit protesters from younger generations who have never known a world without safe, legal abortions, the anti-choice forces have escalated their efforts. Inform yourself about current legal restrictions, mass protests, and harassment of abortion clinic staff and patients by using the following resources:

To Support Reproductive Rights Organizations:

NARAL Pro-Choice America
www.prochoiceamerica.org or 202-973-3000
NARAL Pro-Choice America's mission is to develop and sustain a constituency that uses the political process to guarantee every woman the right to make personal decisions

regarding the full range of reproductive choices, including preventing unintended pregnancy, bearing healthy children, and choosing legal abortion. It is a national organization with affiliates in many states. The website can direct you to more sources of information and action.

To Find Facts from Reliable Sources:

The Guttmacher Institute

www.guttmacher.org

The Guttmacher Institute is a nonprofit organization focused on sexual and reproductive health research, policy analysis, and public education. It is a respected resource with the highest standards in research and reporting.

To Help Someone Who Doesn't Have the Resources to Pay for an Abortion:

Pro-Choice Resources

www.prochoiceresources.org or 612-825-2000

Pro-Choice Resources (PCR) has helped hundreds of women. Its programs are some of the most unique in the country. It is a homegrown nonprofit, not affiliated with any national program. PCR is not a clinic or a lobbying organization and receives no government or United Way funding. It is the only organization in the country to offer education, advocacy, financial assistance, and outreach under one roof. PCR is located in Minnesota, but its programs reach people across the globe. PCR administers the Hersey Abortion Assistance Fund (toll free: 1-888-439-0124) to assist teens and women from across the country with no-interest loans, grants, and resources for those who choose abortion but are unable to afford one. Pro-Choice Resources does extensive education and community outreach to help prevent unwanted pregnancies. Their education website for teens (www.birdsandbees.org) is used by youth from as far away as Israel and Germany.

The National Network of Abortion Funds
www.nnaf.org or 617-524-6040

The National Network of Abortion Funds is one of the best resources for women needing financial help. It provides information for women across the country, helping them find an appropriate fund. You can donate to a specific fund in your area and know the money will go directly to women in need.

To Find Information on Legal Considerations in the United States and around the World:

The Center for Reproductive Rights
www.reproductiverights.org

The Center for Reproductive Rights (formerly the Center for Reproductive Law and Policy) is a nonprofit legal advocacy organization that uses the law to advance reproductive freedom as a fundamental right that all governments are obligated to protect, respect, and fulfill. Founded in 1992, the Center has defined the course of reproductive rights law in the United States with significant legal victories. Using international human rights law, the Center has strengthened reproductive health laws and policies abroad by working with more than fifty organizations in forty-four countries in Africa, Asia, East Central Europe, Latin America, and the Caribbean.

For General Information about Abortion and Reproductive Health:

Citizens Development Corps
www.cdc.org
Citizens Development Corps is a government organization with a wide variety of information on all aspects of health.

Planned Parenthood Federation of America
www.plannedparenthood.org
Planned Parenthood is dedicated to providing information related to family planning for women and men of all ages. An excellent resource.

The Feminist Majority Foundation
www.feminist.org
The Feminist Majority Foundation works for social, political, and economic equality for women by using research and education to improve women's lives.